Department of Veterans Affairs
Health Services Research & Development Service | Evidence-based Synthesis Program

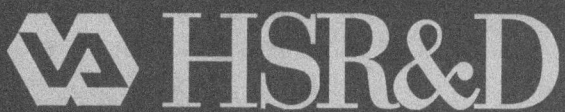

I0470678

A Comparison of Joint Replacement Disparities in VA and Non-VA Settings: A Systematic Review

September 2011

Prepared for:

Department of Veterans Affairs
Veterans Health Administration
Health Services Research & Development Service
Washington, DC 20420

Prepared by:

Evidence-based Synthesis Program (ESP) Center
West Los Angeles VA Medical Center
Los Angeles, CA
Paul G. Shekelle, MD, PhD, Director

Investigators:

Principal Investigators:
   Walid F. Gellad, MD, MPH
   Melinda Maggard Gibbons, MD, MSHS

Research Associates:
   Isomi M. Miake-Lye, BA

Medical Editor:
   Mary E. Vaiana, PhD

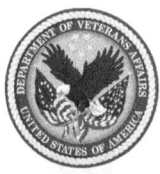

PREFACE

Health Services Research & Development Service's (HSR&D's) Evidence-based Synthesis Program (ESP) was established to provide timely and accurate syntheses of targeted healthcare topics of particular importance to Veterans Affairs (VA) managers and policymakers, as they work to improve the health and healthcare of Veterans. The ESP disseminates these reports throughout VA.

HSR&D provides funding for four ESP Centers and each Center has an active VA affiliation. The ESP Centers generate evidence syntheses on important clinical practice topics, and these reports help:

- develop clinical policies informed by evidence,
- guide the implementation of effective services to improve patient outcomes and to support VA clinical practice guidelines and performance measures, and
- set the direction for future research to address gaps in clinical knowledge.

In 2009, the ESP Coordinating Center was created to expand the capacity of HSR&D Central Office and the four ESP sites by developing and maintaining program processes. In addition, the Center established a Steering Committee comprised of HSR&D field-based investigators, VA Patient Care Services, Office of Quality and Performance, and Veterans Integrated Service Networks (VISN) Clinical Management Officers. The Steering Committee provides program oversight, guides strategic planning, coordinates dissemination activities, and develops collaborations with VA leadership to identify new ESP topics of importance to Veterans and the VA healthcare system.

Comments on this evidence report are welcome and can be sent to Nicole Floyd, ESP Coordinating Center Program Manager, at nicole.floyd@va.gov.

Recommended citation: Gellad WF, Maggard MA, Miake-Lye IM, Shekelle PG. A Comparison of Joint Replacement Disparities in VA and Non-VA Settings: A Systematic Review. VA-ESP Project #05-226; 2011

This report is based on research conducted by the Evidence-based Synthesis Program (ESP) Center located at the West Los Angeles VA Medical Center, Los Angeles, CA funded by the Department of Veterans Affairs, Veterans Health Administration, Office of Research and Development, Health Services Research and Development. The findings and conclusions in this document are those of the author(s) who are responsible for its contents; the findings and conclusions do not necessarily represent the views of the Department of Veterans Affairs or the United States government. Therefore, no statement in this article should be construed as an official position of the Department of Veterans Affairs. No investigators have any affiliations or financial involvement (e.g., employment, consultancies, honoraria, stock ownership or options, expert testimony, grants or patents received or pending, or royalties) that conflict with material presented in the report.

TABLE OF CONTENTS

TABLES

FIGURES

EXECUTIVE SUMMARY

The purpose of this systematic review was to compare what is known about disparities in total joint replacement (TJR) surgery in VA settings with disparities in civilian health care settings.

BACKGROUND

The leading cause of disability in the United States is osteoarthritis. There is no known cure. Consequently, osteoarthritis is managed with a variety of treatments to reduce disability, improve function, and alleviate symptoms. When conservative treatments fail, surgical intervention is indicated. The most effective surgical option for moderate to severe osteoarthritis in the knee or hip is total joint replacement (TJR). TJR is often considered appropriate in cases where other non-surgical treatments have not brought adequate relief. TJR in the management of end-stage osteoarthritis is widely utilized and is considered the fastest growing elective surgery in the nation, if not the world.

Although TJR is highly successful at treating advanced kip or knee osteoarthritis, there is substantial evidence that disparities exist in TJR utilization in non-VA settings, with racial and ethnic disparities being the most documented. This report compares what is known about disparities in TJR in the VA context with disparities in non-VA settings.

The review focused on three key questions:

Key Question #1: What is the evidence about the existence and magnitude of disparities in joint replacement surgery in VA? How does this compare to published studies from non-VA US populations?

Key Question #2: What is the evidence about the patient level, provider level, and system level factors that contribute to disparities in joint replacement surgery in VA? How does this compare to published studies from non-VA populations?

Key Question #3: What is the evidence regarding VA or non-VA interventions to reduce disparities in joint replacement surgery?

METHODS

We searched PubMed from 1966 through July 2011 using standard search terms. We limited the search to PubMed articles involving human subjects and published in the English language. Titles, abstracts, and articles were reviewed in duplicate by physicians trained in the critical analysis of literature. We used a standardized screening form to screen abstracts and a data abstraction form to extract data from full articles. All data were narratively summarized.

Data about study characteristics, patient characteristics, and outcomes were extracted by a trained research associate under the supervision of the Principal Investigators--one a general surgeon, the other a general internist. Both are experienced reviewers. We assessed study quality for clinical trials using the Jadad criteria, and used a modified version of the Newcastle Ottawa Scale (NOS) for non-randomized studies.

DATA SYNTHESIS

We constructed evidence tables showing key study and patient characteristics, methodological quality, and outcomes. We analyzed studies to compare their characteristics, methods, and findings. We compiled a summary of findings for each question based on qualitative synthesis of the findings.

PEER REVIEW

A draft version of this report was reviewed by seven technical experts, as well as by VA clinical leadership. We addressed reviewer comments and incorporated our responses in the final report (Appendix E).

RESULTS

We screened 299 titles, rejected 155, and performed a more detailed review on 144 articles. From these, we identified 75 articles that addressed one or more of the key questions: 25 addressed key question #1, 38 addressed key question #2, and one addressed key question #3.

Key Question #1

What is the evidence about the existence and magnitude of disparities in joint replacement surgery in VA? How does this compare to published studies from non-VA US populations?

Data supporting existence of disparities in joint replacement surgery in VA are not very robust because they come from just three studies, two of which focus on racial disparities and one of which focuses on gender disparities. The magnitude of the racial disparities in VA as documented in these studies is about the same as the magnitude based on more extensive data from non-VA US populations (about 1.5-3 fold). The quality of evidence for this conclusion is low, based on sparseness and age of data. Thus we expect further research, both into racial and gender disparities, to have an important impact on our estimate of the magnitude of disparities.

The literature on racial disparities in total joint replacement outside the VA is more robust than within the VA. Studies of non-VA US populations consistently find that black patients receive fewer total knee replacement (TKR) operations than whites, and men receive fewer TKR operations than women. The quality of evidence for this conclusion is high; thus future research is unlikely to change our confidence about the estimate of effect. However, future research is still necessary to evaluate these disparities over time and assess whether they are increasing or decreasing.

There are fewer studies that examine whether differences in TKR rates represent true disparities based on clinical need. Those that have examined this issue conclude in general, but not consistently, that there are disparities based on clinical need between blacks and nonblacks. The quality of evidence for this conclusion is moderate. Further research is likely to affect our confidence in the estimate of disparities and may change the estimate.

Data about differences in utilization and disparities for total hip replacement in both non-VA US and VA populations are scant, and no conclusions can be drawn. The quality of evidence is therefore very low.

Data about differences in utilization for other races (Hispanic, Asian) are scant, and no conclusions can be drawn. The quality of evidence is therefore very low.

Key Question #2

What is the evidence about the patient level, provider level, and system level factors that contribute to disparities in joint replacement surgery in VA? How does this evidence compare to published studies from non-VA populations?

Only three studies combine both VA and non-VA patients and examine racial disparities in joint replacement, but they are not able to directly compare actual disparities across VA and non-VA sites. In these studies, there were no racial differences in clinical appropriateness for TJR or differences in perceived arthritis severity or susceptibility for worsening. African American patients were less likely than whites to perceive benefits of and more likely to recognize barriers to TJR. There was no difference in clinical appropriateness for patients at a county hospital compared with patients at a nearby VA. Studies found that County hospital patients were nearly 3-fold more likely to be referred to a surgeon compared with VA patients, but this association was not significant when self-reported referral data were used. The quality of evidence for this conclusion is low because all data came from a single cohort, and replication of the results in other patient populations is needed in order to have stronger confidence in the conclusion.

Evidence about the patient-, provider-, and system- level factors that contribute to disparities in joint replacement surgery in the VA comes from a series of small studies recruiting patients from one or two VA medical centers. The studies find generally that black patients, compared with whites, have lower expectations about the effectiveness of joint replacement, less familiarity with the procedure, and may be more likely to view prayer and other techniques as useful for managing arthritis pain. There is some evidence that blacks may be less likely to be referred to specialists for joint replacement or to have TJR recommended by a specialist; however, some of these differences may be explained by patient preferences. One study examining communication between patients and orthopedic surgeons in the VA found little difference by race.

Although the individual studies are of high quality, the overall quality of evidence for the above conclusions is low because the studies were small and limited to a few sites. It is also likely that further research into important mediators (such as patient preference) and research with different patient cohorts will have an important impact on conclusions about the reasons for these joint disparities. The age of the data is also a limiting factor: a majority of the studies come from patient cohorts recruited over 10 years ago, and 8 of those studies come from a single VA medical center.

Data about reasons for disparities for other races (Hispanic, Asian) are scant, and no conclusions can be drawn. The quality of evidence is therefore very low.

Evidence in non-VA settings suggests that minority patients (African Americans being the most studied) may have less knowledge about joint replacement surgery, perceive fewer health benefits, and have greater fear about the surgery, similar to findings within VA. These patients may be less likely to be referred to a surgeon and are less likely to consider surgery. When they do present for surgery, African Americans have more advanced disease. Disease severity, socioeconomic factors, or degree of comorbidities do not appear to account for all of these differences. Minority patients may be less likely to be treated in high volume centers or by high volume providers, which is a system-level factor that has not been studied within VA.

Key Question #3

What is the evidence regarding VA or non-VA interventions to reduce disparities in joint replacement surgery?

There has been only one published VA study of an intervention to improve disparities. It focused on expectations and examined only total knee replacement. It found that, after watching an informational video, African Americans, but not Caucasians, had statistically significant improvements in their expectations for pain and function post-operatively. Other potential causes of disparities have not been the subjects of interventions, and no study has yet assessed changes in the actual delivery of joint replacement surgery.

The quality of evidence for this key question is very low, due to sparseness of data; thus any estimate of effect is uncertain.

ABBREVIATIONS TABLE

Table 1. Abbreviations

Abbreviation	Definition
OA	Osteoarthritis
THR	Total Hip Replacement
TKR	Total Knee Replacement
TJR	Total Joint Replacement (TJR is also used for Total Joint Arthroplasty, which is sufficiently similar)

EVIDENCE REPORT

INTRODUCTION

BACKGROUND

The leading cause of disability in the United States is osteoarthritis.[1, 2] There is no known cure. Consequently, osteoarthritis is managed with a variety of treatments to reduce disability, improve function, and alleviate symptoms. The most effective surgical option for moderate to severe osteoarthritis in the knee or hip is total joint replacement (TJR).[3, 4] TJR is often considered appropriate in cases where other non-surgical treatments have not brought adequate relief.[2, 5-7]

Although TJR is highly successful at treating advanced hip or knee osteoarthritis, there is a large body of evidence suggesting that disparities exist in TJR utilization in non-VA settings.[8-19] Although subgroups of patients may utilize services differently depending on clinical needs, Kane et al. explain that "disparity in healthcare implies unequality, unlikeness, or unfair disproportion,"[20] as opposed to extensive accepted variation in practice.[21, 22] Measuring disparities usually means comparing rates of utilization of care, since measuring access to care directly can be difficult.[20] But if only utilization is measured, and need for care is not taken into account, disparities might not be fully characterized. "Need for care" data are not easily captured, making this concept almost as hard to measure as access to care. Utilization data are so often relied upon when discussing disparities because of this difficulty of measuring access to care or need for care.

In order to remedy disparities, they must first be documented and their causes better understood. Disparities in TJR utilizations have been well documented outside VA. The purpose of this report is to compare what is known about disparities in TJR in non-VA settings to disparities in TJR in the VA context.

Our conceptual framework identifies three "generations" of studies of disparities, based on whether the studies are documenting disparities, examining their underlying reasons, or assessing interventions to address them (see Figure 1).

Figure 1. Conceptual Framework

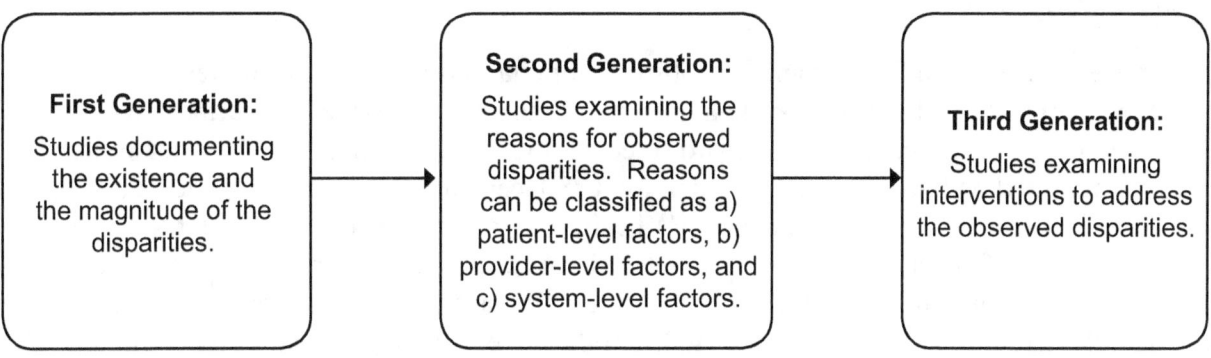

METHODS

TOPIC DEVELOPMENT

This project was nominated by Tamara L. Martin, MD and the Center for Health Equity Research and Promotion, with input from a technical expert group that included Said Ibrahim and David Atkins.

The final key questions are:

Key Question #1. What is the evidence about the existence and magnitude of disparities in joint replacement surgery in VA? How does this compare to published studies from non-VA US populations?

Key Question #2: What is the evidence about the patient level, provider level, and system level factors that contribute to disparities in joint replacement surgery in VA? How does this compare to published studies from non-VA populations?

Key Question #3: What is the evidence regarding VA or non-VA interventions to reduce disparities in joint replacement surgery?

Evidence Synthesis Program systematic reviews are done according to a standard protocol, which is modeled on the protocol used by the Evidence-Based Practice Center program. A detailed individual protocol is not created for each separate topic.

SEARCH STRATEGY

We searched PubMed for relevant literature from 1966 through July 2011, using standard search terms such as "disparities," "variations," "replacement," and "arthroplasty" (see Appendix A for complete search strategy). We limited the search to peer-reviewed articles involving human subjects and published in the English language. We judged it unlikely for studies of US patients, either VA or non-VA, to be published in non-English language journals. Since our focus was US studies, we elected to forgo searching EMBASE. Also, since RCTs are not the study design to assess anything but third generation disparity questions, we elected to forgo searching the Cochrane Central Register of Controlled Trials (CENTRAL).

STUDY SELECTION

Two reviewers assessed for relevance the abstracts of citations identified from literature searches. Full text articles of potentially relevant abstracts were retrieved for further review. Each article was reviewed using a standard screener form (see Appendix B). Inclusion criteria were: 1) reported on hip, knee (or both) total joint replacement; 2) reported on patients treated within the VA or who were treated in non-VA health care settings in the United States; and 3) reported results of either racial/ethnic or gender disparities. There were no inclusion or exclusion criteria for study design. We excluded studies of joint replacement surgery for other sites (such as shoulder). Additionally, we excluded studies if there were about gender differences in the technical approach to the procedure (e.g., use of gender-specific prostheses).

DATA ABSTRACTION

We abstracted the following data for each included study for the key questions: intervention(s), data source, study subjects, patient selection, years of data collection, study design, outcome measure(s), categorization of race(s), determination of race, assessment of receipt of procedure, assessment of disparity outcome, population sample size, mean/median patient age, response rate, subject follow-up, and covariates for result adjustment (Appendix C).

QUALITY ASSESSMENT

We assessed individual randomized studies using the criteria of Jadad.[23] We assessed non-randomized studies using items taken or derived from the Newcastle Ottawa Scale, involving representativeness of the sample and how key variables were assessed[24] (see Appendix D for adapted variables).

DATA SYNTHESIS

We constructed evidence tables showing the study characteristics and results for all included studies, organized by key question. We critically analyzed studies to compare their characteristics, methods, and findings. We compiled a summary of findings for each key question or clinical topic, and drew conclusions based on qualitative synthesis of the findings. We used the conceptual framework of Kilbourne and colleagues (see Figure 2) to organize the reasons for disparities assessed in the second-generation studies.[25]

Figure 2. Kilbourne et al. model:[25] Understanding the origins of health and health care disparities from a health services research perspective: key potential determinants of health disparities within the health care system, including individual, provider, and health care system factors

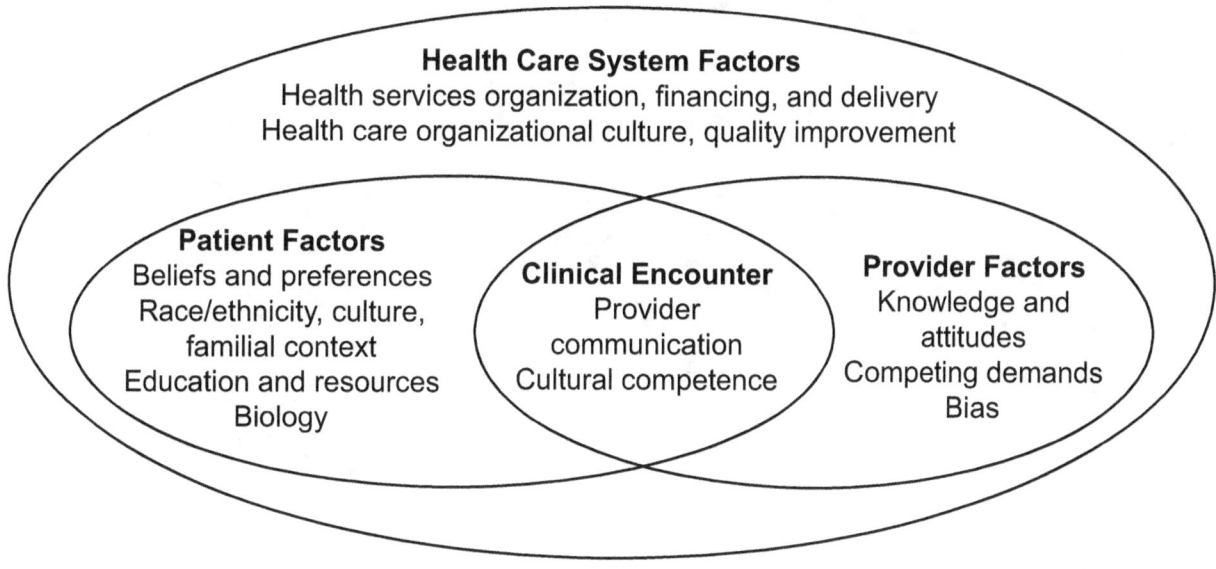

RATING THE BODY OF EVIDENCE

We assessed the overall quality of evidence for outcomes using a method developed by the GRADE Working Group, which classified the evidence across outcomes according to the following criteria:

- High = Further research is very unlikely to change our confidence about the estimate of effect.
- Moderate = Further research is likely to have an important impact on our confidence in the estimate of effect and may change the estimate.
- Low = Further research is very likely to have an important impact on our confidence in the estimate of effect and is likely to change the estimate.
- Very Low = Any estimate of effect is very uncertain.

The ESP SharePoint site {http://vaww.infoshare.va.gov/sites/hsrd/esp/default.aspx} contains reference articles that describe guidelines for the GRADE quality assessment system.

PEER REVIEW

A draft version of this report was reviewed by seven technical experts as well as by VA clinical leadership. Their comments and our responses are presented in Appendix E.

RESULTS

LITERATURE FLOW

Our literature search identified 284 titles and abstracts from the electronic search, and one additional article from reference mining, for a total of 285 references. We excluded 155 titles as being clearly irrelevant. We conducted an update search after peer review, which yielded 12 new articles, with an additional two articles from reference mining, bringing the total up to 299 references. We retrieved 144 full-text articles for further review and excluded another 70 references for various reasons (see Figure 3). We identified a total of 74 references for inclusion in the current review. We grouped the studies by key question, type of disparity, and whether the patient population was of VA or non-VA origin. Figure 3 details the flow of articles from citations to the number of references informing each of the key questions.

Figure 3. Literature Flow

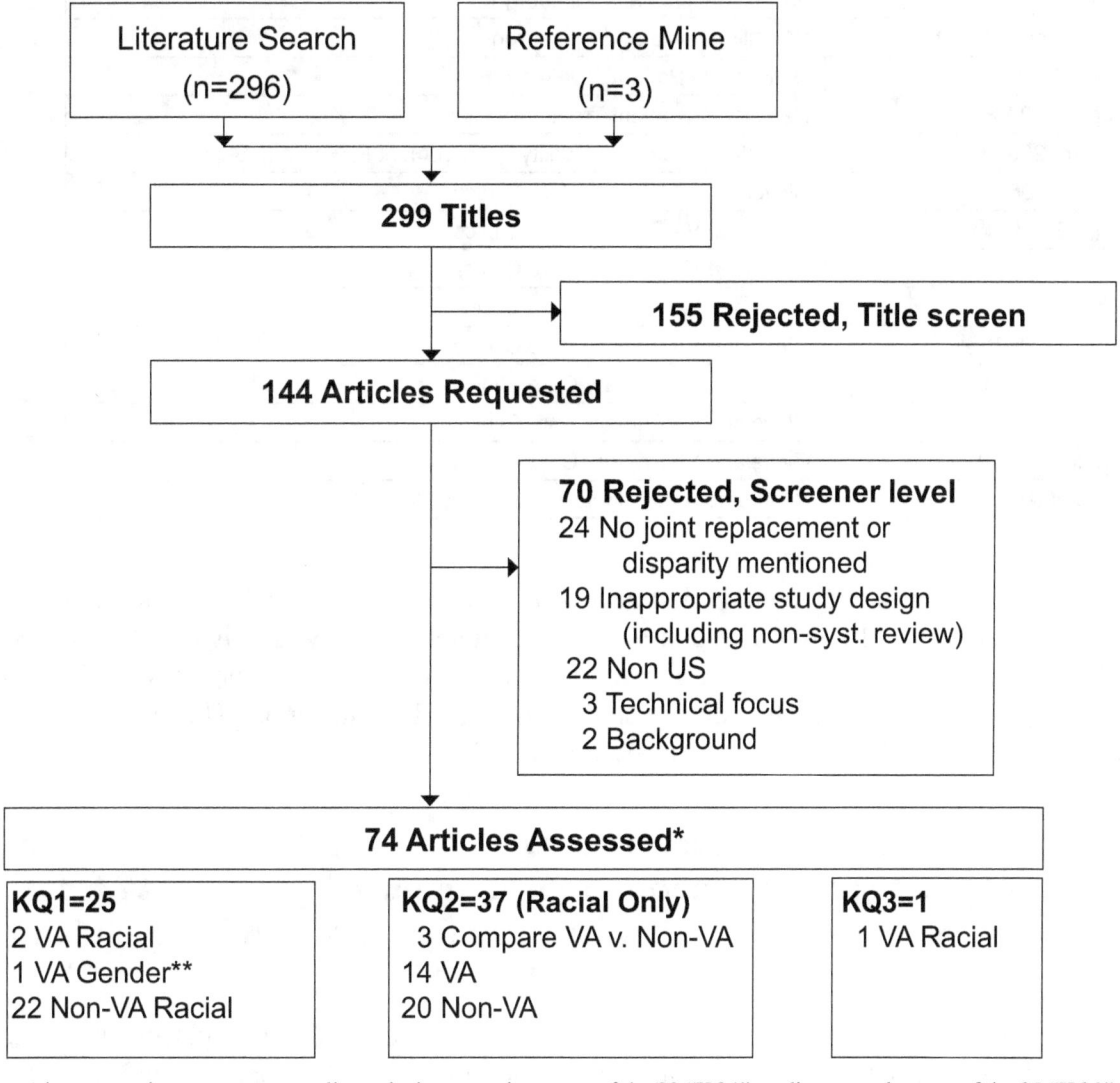

*Key question categories were not mutually exclusive, meaning some of the 22 "KQ1" studies were also part of the 35 "KQ2" category.

**The 28 articles addressing gender disparities in non-VA populations were not included in the tables or report.

DESCRIPTION OF EVIDENCE

Studies of racial disparities in joint replacement that focus on VA patients are clustered around 7 patient cohorts (see Table 2). Two of these studies report on rates of receipt of total joint replacement (first generation studies[26, 27]); the remaining are second generation studies attempting to identify mechanisms underlying the known disparities. One study[28] includes Hispanic ethnicity; otherwise the studies focus on disparities between blacks and whites.

Table 2. Cohort description

Author/year	Study Cohort
Hausmann, 2010[26]	Orthopedic Clinics Pittsburgh and Cleveland
Hausmann, 2011[29]	Orthopedic Clinics Pittsburgh and Cleveland
Ang, 2009[30]	VA+ County Hospital in Indiana
Ang, 2009[31]	VA+ County Hospital in Indiana
Ang, 2008[32]	VA+ County Hospital in Indiana
Jones, 2008[33]	VA Philadelphia and Pittsburgh
Groeneveld, 2008[34]	VA Philadelphia and Pittsburgh
Jones, 2005[27]	National VA Patient Treatment Files
Borrero, 2006[35]	National VA Patient Treatment Files
Ibrahim, 2005[28]	VA National Surgical Quality Improvement Program (NSQIP)
Lopez, 2005[36]	Cleveland VA Primary Care Clinics
Ang, 2003[37]	Cleveland VA Primary Care Clinics
Ibrahim, 2003[38]	Cleveland VA Primary Care Clinics
Ibrahim, 2002[39]	Cleveland VA Primary Care Clinics
Ibrahim, 2002[40]	Cleveland VA Primary Care Clinics
Ibrahim, 2002[41]	Cleveland VA Primary Care Clinics
Ibrahim, 2002[42]	Cleveland VA Primary Care Clinics
Ibrahim, 2001[43]	Cleveland VA Primary Care Clinics
Weng 2007[44]	VA Greater Los Angeles Ambulatory Care

In addition we identified 22 non-VA first generation studies, one of which was a systematic review.[20] There were 21 non-VA second-generation studies. There was only one third-generation study, which was of VA patients. For gender disparities, we identified 29 non-VA studies and one VA (first-generation) study. Only the VA study is discussed in this report. The evidence tables present details of each included study (see Appendix F).

KEY QUESTION #1. What is the evidence about the existence and magnitude of disparities in joint replacement surgery in VA? How does this compare to published studies from non-VA US populations?

VA Data

Three first-generation studies report on disparities in receipt of total joint replacement in VA settings. Two studies used national data; one was based in two institutions. All three studies were judged to have population-based or otherwise representative patient samples. Race was identified using self-report in one study and administrative data in the other two. In all three studies, administrative or medical record data were used to determine if a procedure had been performed. In all three studies, response rate or adequacy of follow-up were not applicable (see Appendix F, evidence table 1).

One study examines a local cohort of 457 veterans seen between 2005-2008;[26] another uses national VA patient treatment files from 1999-2001 to report on rates of receipt of knee replacement (only) among 260,856 veterans.[27] Hausmann et al.[26] recruited patients immediately before and after their orthopedic surgery clinic visit at two large VA hospitals (Pittsburgh and Cleveland) between 2005 and 2008. The primary outcome was whether patients received a recommendation for TJR from the surgeon, as determined by electronic medical record review. The secondary outcome was receipt of TJR at the VA within 6 months of study enrollment. The odds of receiving a TJR recommendation were lower for blacks than for white patients of similar age and disease severity (OR 0.46, 95% CI 0.26-0.83). This difference, however, was no longer significant after adjusting for patient preference for TJR (measured using a single item question). The adjusted odds of actual receipt of TJR were lower for blacks than for whites, although the results did not reach statistical significance (OR 0.41, 95% CI 0.16-1.05).

In the second first-generation study, Jones et al.[27] examine 260,856 patients with osteoarthritis (based on ICD-9 code 715.x) from the national VA patient treatment files in 1999 with 2-year follow up to determine rates of TKR. In the final statistical model, adjusting for age, gender, and Charlson comorbidity (without adjustment for disease severity), black patients were less likely than whites to have received TKR (OR 0.72, 95% CI 0.65-0.80).

One of the three studies reporting on disparities in receipt of TJR in VA settings assessed gender disparities.[45] Borrero and colleagues analyzed a national sample of 1,986,093 VA patients aged 50 years or older (1,923,524 male, 44,569 female) in the VA National Patient Care Database during fiscal year 1999. In this cohort, 172 (0.4%) women and 5,198 (0.3%) men received TKR (P<.001), and 91 (0.2%) women and 2,618 (0.1%) men received THR (P=.001). The odds ratios for receipt of TJR was 1.4 for women compared to men, which demonstrated the statistically significantly higher rates of TKR and THR in women. However, after adjusting for the presence of OA, there was no longer any significant difference in odds of receipt of TJR. The authors noted that women have a higher prevalence of OA-related disability, and additionally adjusted for this in an OA subcohort of 329,461 patients (319,924 male, 9,537 female), which consisted of patients with a diagnosis of OA using the ICD-9-CM code. Within this subcohort, there were no differences by gender: 153 (1.6%) women and 4,638 (1.5%) men had TKR, and 73 (0.8%) women and 2147 (0.7%) men had THR. The authors suggest that an important factor in understanding gender differences in TJR is the difference in OA prevalence between men and women.

Non-VA Data

The literature on racial disparities in total joint replacement outside the VA is more robust than within the VA. However, we found only one systematic review on the topic of disparities in total knee replacement (Kane et al.[20]). An additional review on the epidemiology of knee and hip arthroplasty was identified.[19] Its focus was not on disparities, nevertheless data on differences in utilization by gender and race was reported.

In 2007, Kane et al.[20] published the results of a systematic review examining disparities in total knee replacement performed by the Minnesota Evidence-Based Practice Center and commissioned by the Agency for Healthcare Research and Quality. The review was presented to experts at an NIH Consensus Conference on Total Knee Replacement in December 2003. In discussing the limitations of the literature, the authors mention that some of the studies address rates of procedure use without paying attention to the size of the population at risk (patients with severe symptomatic knee/hip OA who might have an indication for TJR); this limitation is worth noting as rates of use are presented below.

The authors limited their search to English language articles between 1995-2003 and excluded studies with less than 100 observations; of the 176 references that they identified, only 4 met the inclusion criteria. The authors added another 3 studies from reference mining, for a total of 7 studies. The 7 studies primarily use Medicare national claims to examine rates of disparities, with the exception of two studies: one examined a community cohort of elderly patients with arthritis, and the other examined a cross-sectional survey of people age 55 or older in Ontario, Canada. Each of the studies finds the highest rates of TKR use in whites compared with nonwhites. Most of these studies examining gender disparities found that women were more likely to receive joint replacement than men; in one study,[46] women were less likely to receive joint replacement after adjusting for presence and severity of arthritis. The results of the Kane and colleagues review indicate that there are racial/ethnic and gender disparities in the receipt of TKR in the United States.

A recent systematic review by Singh[19] focused on studies of the incidence and prevalence of knee and hip arthroplasty. Included in this review were data from six studies, three of them from the United States, all reporting differences in utilization rates by gender, ethnicity, or both.

Our search found nine overlapping references that will not be discussed further, as they were included in Kane or Singh.[8, 11, 12, 16, 47-51] Although not discussed here, they still appear in the evidence tables (see Appendix F).

More recent studies document the continued existence of racial/ethnic disparities in TKR. Jha et al.[52] describe rates of both TKR and THR among the Medicare fee for service population, this time comparing 1992 to 2001. In their analysis, they compare blacks vs. nonblack patients in Medicare and stratified the analysis by gender. In each analysis, women had higher age-adjusted rates of procedure use than men, and nonblacks had higher rates than blacks. In 2001, nonblack men had a rate of 5.05/1000 population for TKR, compared with 1.85 for black men. Among women, rates of TKR per 1000 population were 6.6 among nonblacks and 5.1 among blacks.

In another analysis of Medicare (one of the few including Hispanic ethnicity) from 2000, Skinner et al.[53] compare rates of TKR adjusted for age and income and find that, compared with white men, the odds ratio for receipt of TKR for black men was 0.36 (0.34,0.38), for Hispanic men 0.67 (0.62-0.73), and for Asian men 0.28 (0.24,0.32). White women and Hispanic women were more likely and as likely, respectively, as white men to receive TKR.

Another study looked at Medigap coverage and found disparities in receipt of joint replacement based on whether patients lived in a high, standard or low minority area. Patients were defined as living in a high-minority area if 60% or more of the population in their zip code was in one of the nonwhite minority groups. Low minority area was defined as 15% or less of residents in one of the non-white minority groups. Patients living in high minority areas were 20% less likely to undergo a hip or knee replacement as those who resided in low minority areas.[54]

Four additional studies, using older data and non-Medicare data sources, also found significant disparities. In an analysis using the Nationwide Inpatient Sample from 1990-2000, Jain et al.[55] examine the percentage of all TKRs performed on black patients vs. white patients; however, the overall rate of TKR among blacks and whites is not known, and 27% of race data was missing. They found that the percentage of all TKRs performed on black patients has increased from 1990-1993 (4.2% black), to 1994-1998 (5.9% black), to 1998-2000 (6.5% black).

Bang also used the Nationwide Inpatient Sample, but from 1996-2005, and found that non-white groups had lower odds of THA and TKA compared with whites.[56] All racial minority groups were 23% to 64% less likely to undergo arthroplasties. Racial disparities were larger than income disparities, and racial disparities were not confined to elderly or to low-income.

Hanchate et al.[57] describe rates of knee replacement in the Health and Retirement Survey (HRS) from 1994-2004. They find no racial/ethnic differences in rates of TKR among women after adjusting for economic factors, including insurance, income, assets, and age. However, they find that black men are significantly less likely than white women to receive a TKR (OR 0.56 (0.33-0.95), although the difference is no longer statistically significant when the sample is limited to those with self-reported arthritis. There were no disparities comparing Hispanics and whites.

Finally, an analysis using hospital discharge data from Connecticut from 1996-1998, Olson and Foland[58] examined rates of TKR; the analysis did not account for rates of severe OA, or preferences or need for TKR. They found that the age adjusted rates per 100K discharges for TKR was highest for black women (115.8, 95% CI 103.9-127.7) and lowest for black men (44, 34.9-68.9) and Hispanic men (16.9, 10.1-23.8) and women (47.5, 37.8-57.2). White women had rates of 84.9 (82.4-87.4) and white men 66.5 (63.9 -68.9).

The Kane review focused on total knee replacement. There are no systematic reviews specifically examining racial/ethnic disparities in total hip replacement (THR). Many of the studies examining hip replacement use data that are quite old. Jha et al.[52] included hip replacement in their analyses of Medicare data and found that in 2001, nonblack men had a rate of THR of 2.60/1000 population compared with 1.08/1000 for blacks. Among women, rates per 1000 population in THR were 3.33 for nonblacks and 1.86 for blacks. Using data from 1997-2001 hospital discharge records from two states included in the HCUP, Basu and Mobley[59] found no difference in the likelihood of THR between blacks, whites and Hispanics in either 1997 or 2000, after adjusting for income, urban/rural, distance from hospital, and social isolation. They did not adjust for severity of arthritis.

Two older studies (from the 1980s) using hospital discharge records from Hawaii[60] and California[14] examined rates of THR; the studies did not include information about the need for the procedure. Oishi et al.[60] found no differences in rates of THR among whites and Asians for those under age 50, but lower rates among Asians for those over age of 50. Giacomini[14] found no statistically significant difference in THR rates after adjusting for insurance status, age and comorbidities between whites, Hispanics, and blacks; however, Asians had lower odds of THR (0.47, 0.29-0.77).

One study outside the VA examined disparities in joint replacement surgery, combining TKR and THR. Francis et al.[61] reported rates of TKR/THR in 2005 Medicare data, comparing rural and urban beneficiaries. They found that nonwhites are less likely than whites in rural areas to receive joint replacement (OR 0.69, 0.66-0.71); the disparity is more pronounced in urban areas. African Americans had lower odds than whites for receipt of the procedures in rural areas (OR 0.68, 0.65-0.71). There were no differences in adjusted rates of joint replacement for Hispanic vs. white in rural areas, but there were differences in urban areas (OR 0.62).

Finally, in one of the few studies that examined rates of TKR/THR among those in need (based on difficulty walking, joint pain, stiffness, or swelling),[62] African American patients in the Health and Retirement Study (HRS) from 1998-2004 were less likely to receive joint replacement than whites (OR 0.34 (0.17-0.66)). The higher rate of joint replacement in women compared to men was appropriate, based on their assessment of need.

Summary of Findings

Data supporting existence of disparities in joint replacement surgery in VA are not very robust because they come from just three studies, two of which focus on racial disparities and only one of which focuses on gender disparities The magnitude of the racial disparities in VA as documented in these studies is about the same as the magnitude based on more extensive data from non-VA US populations (about 1.5-3 fold). The quality of evidence for this conclusion is low, based on sparseness and age of data. Thus we expect further research, both into racial and gender disparities, to have an important impact on our estimate of the magnitude of disparities.

The literature on racial disparities in total joint replacement outside the VA is more robust than within the VA. Studies of non-VA US populations consistently find that black patients receive fewer TKR operations than whites, and men receive fewer TKR operations than women. The quality of evidence for this conclusion is high; thus future research is unlikely to change our confidence about the estimate of effect. However, future research is still necessary to evaluate these disparities over time and assess whether they are increasing or decreasing.

There are fewer studies that examine whether differences in TKR rates represent true disparities based on clinical need. Those that have examined this issue conclude in general, but not consistently, that disparities in joint replacement between blacks and non-blacks persist after adjusting for clinical need. The quality of evidence for this conclusion is moderate. Further research is likely to affect our confidence in the estimate of disparities and may change the estimate.

Data about differences in utilization and disparities for total hip replacement in both non-VA US and VA populations are scant, and no conclusions can be drawn. The quality of evidence is therefore very low.

Data about differences in utilization for other races (Hispanic, Asian) are scant, and no conclusions can be drawn. The quality of evidence is therefore very low.

KEY QUESTION #2. What is the evidence about the patient level, provider level, and system level factors that contribute to disparities in joint replacement surgery in VA? How does this compare to published studies from non-VA populations?

Direct Comparison of VA and Non-VA Patients

Three studies include both VA and non-VA patients and examine racial disparities in joint replacement, thus potentially providing the most direct comparison between VA and non VA.[30-32] These three papers, however, report on the same cohort of patients and are not able to compare actual disparities across VA and non-VA patients, since site of care is used primarily as an adjustment variable. Patients were collected from one prospective study of primary care clinics that referred patients to a VA medical center (serving Indiana and surrounding states) and from patients in a non-VA County hospital, which was near the VA, with primary care network and community health care centers (Indianapolis). Race was self-reported.

The primary outcomes of interest were racial disparities in clinical appropriateness, perceived health beliefs of TJR, and referral to an orthopedic surgeon. Outcomes were assessed using the medical record and self-report. The sample size varied slightly between reports, ranging from 676 to 691. Approximately 90% of eligible subjects participated. The patient cohort comprised 38% African Americans (AA) and 72% whites, all of whom had at least moderate osteoarthritis. Eligibility criteria included age (>50 y/o), radiographic evidence of osteoarthritis, and Western Ontario and McMaster Universities Osteoarthritis Index (WOMAC) summary score >=30. There were differences in the racial distribution of patients by recruitment site: 64% of the African American patients and 30% of whites were recruited from the county hospital

Results showed no differences in clinical appropriateness for TJR between the racial groups: (appropriate for TJR: 25.5% AA versus 29.4% whites; inappropriate: 74.5% AA versus 70.6% whites; P=0.3).[31] Multivariate regression confirmed that race did not predict clinical appropriateness (OR=1.2 [0.8–1.8]; P=0.3). Clinical appropriateness was determined using an algorithm based on 5 variables: adequacy of medical management, WOMAC pain severity, WOMAC functional limitation, age (50–70 years or >70 years), and medical comorbidity. Patients were categorized as appropriate, uncertain, or inappropriate for TJR. Appropriate represented a patient who was severely symptomatic (pain and function) despite medical management, and could undergo surgery with acceptable risk. This validated algorithm show that appropriateness was associated with better health-related quality of life following TJR. There was no difference in clinical appropriateness between county and VA patients (28.8% versus 27.2%, P=0.6).

A similar analysis of 684 patients from this cohort looked at the association of race with health beliefs and barriers to TJR.[32] This outcome was assessed using the modified Arthritis-related Health Belief Instrument (AHBI), based on the Health Belief Model. AHBI reports 4 themes: perceived arthritis severity, perceived susceptibility for arthritis to worsen, perceived benefits of arthroplasty, and perceived barriers to arthroplasty. This analysis identified differences in health beliefs and barriers to TJR. African American patients were less likely than whites to perceive benefits of TJR (OR=.60 [.42-.86]; P=.005) and more likely to recognize barriers to TJR (OR=1.7 [1.18-2.44]; P=.004). The analysis did not find any racial differences in perceived arthritis severity or susceptibility that arthritis would worsen. Recruitment site was predictive of perceived benefits of TJR: County patients were less likely than VA patients to perceive benefits of TJR (OR=.45 [.23-.89]; P=0.02). Hospital site (county versus VA) did not predict perception of barriers to THR (OR=1.38 [0.71-2.66]; P=.33). Race and hospital site interactions were not significant.

The third study assessed the same patient cohort (n=676); the primary outcome was referral to an orthopedic surgeon.[30] Race, clinical appropriateness, and health beliefs were included in the analyses. Neither race (HR=1.39 [0.94–2.05]; P=0.1) nor any of the four health belief themes (HR range 0.99 to 1.05) predicted referral to a surgeon. However, clinical appropriateness did predict referral (HR=1.95 [1.15-3.32]; P=0.01). Regression models controlled for recruitment site (county versus VA). In a univariate analysis, non-VA patients were more likely to be referred to an orthopedic surgeon than were VA patients (60.5% compared with 39.5%, P<0.0001). Multivariate regression showed that county patients were more likely (HR=2.7 [1.4 –5.1], P=0.0026) than the VA patients to be referred to surgery. Interactions of race with hospital site, health beliefs, and clinical appropriateness were not significant.

Summary of Findings

Only three studies combine both VA and non-VA patients and examine racial disparities in joint replacement, but they are not able to directly compare actual disparities across VA and non-VA sites. There were no racial differences in clinical appropriateness for TJR or differences in perceived arthritis severity or susceptibility for worsening. African American patients were less likely than whites to perceive benefits of and more likely to recognize barriers to TJR. There was no difference in clinical appropriateness for patients at a county hospital compared with patients at a nearby VA. Studies found that County hospital patients were nearly 3-fold more likely to be referred to a surgeon compared with VA patients, but this association was not significant when self-reported referral data were used. The quality of evidence for this conclusion is low because all data came from a single cohort, and replication of the results in other patient populations is needed in order to have stronger confidence in the conclusion.

VA Data

Each of the additional studies of joint replacement in VA comes from one of the other 6 patient cohorts, as described above (Table 2). All but one are small studies of patients in either one or two VA Medical Centers; the larger study used NSQIP data.[28] Two studies had population-based or otherwise representative sampling of patients; the rest used convenience samples. Race was identified by self report except for the larger study, which used administrative data. Assessment of receipt of the procedure was a criterion that only applied in two of the studies, one using administrative data, the other using medical records. Response rates were not recorded for about half of the studies; in the remainder, response rates were high.

In a majority of cases, the studies focused on patient factors that might explain racial disparities in procedure use, but in a few cases the studies deal with topics that overlap patient, provider, and health system factors as well as the clinical encounter (based on conceptual framework, Figure 2 above).

In one VA cohort, patients aged 50-79 with chronic knee or hip pain and WOMAC score greater than 38 were enrolled from primary care clinics at the Philadelphia and Pittsburgh VA

Medical Centers between 2004 and 2006. The first study from this cohort[33] examined racial differences in the pain coping strategies for 939 of these patients. This analysis found that, of the various coping strategies, blacks relied more on hoping and praying compared with whites (Beta = 0.74, 95% CI 0.50-0.99), and blacks were more likely to view prayer as helpful (OR 3.38, 95% CI 2.35-4.86) and to have tried prayer (OR 2.28, 95% CI 1.66-3.13) to manage their pain. Groeneveld et al.[34] report on a second study using the same cohort to examine racial differences in the expectations of the effectiveness of joint replacement in improving quality of life, measured using a validated survey scale (JRES). After adjusting for disease severity, socioeconomic factors, literacy, and trust, there were small but statistically significant differences in patient expectations, with blacks having lower expectations for both knee and hip OA. The authors note that the clinical and policy significance of these differences is not clear.

Eight of the VA studies on racial disparities in joint replacement come from a cohort of 596 patients from primary care clinics at the Cleveland VA in 1997-2000.[36-43] Participants in the cohort were approached and asked about their hip/knee pain, and they were eligible for inclusion if they self-identified as white or black, were over age 50, and had at least moderate severity symptoms based on the Lequesne OA Severity Index. Each of the studies (which had considerable overlap in authorship) is described in more detail below. All focus on patient factors underlying joint replacement disparities; two also involve the overlap of patient and provider factors and the clinical encounter.

In the earliest study based on this cohort, Ibrahim et al.[43] examined differences in the perceptions of the efficacy of traditional treatments and complementary treatments and self-care practices for osteoarthritis. In adjusted analyses, blacks were less likely to believe that joint replacement was efficacious compared with whites (OR 0.52, 95% CI 0.28-0.98) and were more likely to rely on self-care measures for their arthritis. The same authors published a second study[42] that examined differences in the familiarity and knowledge of respondents about joint replacement within the same cohort; black patients were less likely than white patients to be familiar with joint replacement surgery (had ever heard of TJR or had family/friends with TJR or reported a 'good understanding' of TJR) and more likely to express concerns about post-operative pain and walking ability.

In a third study from the Cleveland VA cohort[41] examining self-assessed quality of life, the same authors found that black race was associated with worsened quality of life; the analyses adjusted for WOMAC score, depression, and other clinical factors. In a fourth study, Ang et al.[40] focused on the 'helpfulness of prayer' in the treatment of OA and how that belief affected attitudes towards arthroplasty. They found that black patients were more likely than whites to perceive prayer as helpful in the management of their arthritis (OR 2.1, 95% CI 1.19-3.72) and were less likely to consider surgery for severe arthritis pain (OR 0.59, 95% CI 0.34-0.99). The authors suggest that feelings about the helpfulness of prayer among black patients may explain part of the differences found in the rates of TJR among patients with osteoarthritis.

Two of the studies from the Cleveland VA cohort[37, 38] describe differences in how pain is perceived between blacks and whites with osteoarthritis. Ang et al.[37] examined differences in perceptions of pain and functional disability between blacks and whites at a given level of radiographic severity of arthritis. They found no differences in mean pain and function scores (from the WOMAC). The authors interpret these findings as evidence that differences in perceived symptoms do not explain the observed disparities in joint replacement. Ibrahim et al.[38] report on an exploratory factor analysis in a subsample of these patients (300 veterans). They find a different factor structure in descriptions of pain among blacks and whites, and note that these descriptions of pain did not correlate with radiologic stage of disease. They suggest that blacks and whites with chronic joint osteoarthritis describe the quality of their pain differently.

Two final studies from this Cleveland cohort of 596 patients focus primarily on outcomes that involve considerable overlap between patient and provider factors and the clinical encounter. Ibrahim et al.[39] report on racial differences in the willingness to consider surgery, familiarity with joint replacement surgery, and outcome expectations among patients with arthritis. Blacks had lower odds of having family/friends with TJR (OR 0.39, 95% CI 0.26-0.61) and lower odds of ever hearing of TJR (OR 0.64, 95% CI 0.37-1.09). They were also more likely than whites to expect a longer hospital course and moderate to severe pain and difficulty walking after TJR. Willingness to consider TJR was assessed using one question: "If your pain were to get severe, would you consider surgery to replace your knee/hip if your doctor recommended it?" After adjusting for demographic characteristics, clinical severity, and familiarity with surgery, blacks were less likely than whites to respond yes (OR 0.53, 95% CI 0.30-0.96). However, after adjusting for outcome expectations, the difference between blacks and whites in willingness to consider TKR was no longer significant (OR 0.86, 95% CI 0.45-1.63). Here the authors suggest that expectations of postsurgical course mediated the differences in willingness to have surgery. Lopez et al.[36] examine referrals to specialists and satisfaction with care among this same cohort of patients with knee and/or hip OA. They find that blacks were less likely to view the quality of the primary care relationship as excellent (24.7% vs. 36.3%, p<.01) and less likely to receive a referral to an orthopedic surgeon (17.4% vs. 24.2%); the latter did not reach statistical significance (p = 0.06). In multivariate analyses adjusted for severity of disease, blacks had lower odds of referral to an orthopedic surgeon (OR 0.61, 95% CI 0.36-1.03), although the relationship only approached statistical significance.

Four additional studies using different VA cohorts examine determinants of disparities in joint replacement that overlap between patient, provider, and clinical factors. In the second VA study using national data from the Veterans Administration National Surgical Quality Improvement Program (NSQIP), and the only study including Hispanic veterans, Ibrahim et al.[28] report on the differences in outcomes between black, white and Hispanic veterans who undergo hip and knee arthroplasty between 1996 and 2000-6,703 patients and 12,108 patients respectively. They examine rates of risk-adjusted 30-day mortality and rates of both infectious and non-infectious complications. There were no racial/ethnic differences in 30-day mortality, although there were differences in complication rates. Black patients had higher infection and non-infection related complications following knee replacement (RR 1.42, 95% CI 1.06-1.90, and 1.50, 95% CI 1.08-2.10, respectively.) Hispanic patients had a higher risk of infection (but not non-infection) related complications compared to whites (RR 1.64, 95% CI 1.08-2.49). There were no racial differences in hip arthroplasty complications.

Hausmann et al.[26, 29] recruited patients immediately before and after their orthopedic surgery clinic visit at two large VA hospitals (Pittsburgh and Cleveland) between 2005 and 2008, and report on two separate studies. In the first,[26] the primary outcome was whether patients received a recommendation for TJR from the surgeon, as determined by electronic medical record review. The authors found the odds of receiving a TJR recommendation were lower for blacks than for white patients of similar age and disease severity (OR 0.46, 95% CI 0.26-0.83); however, the difference was no longer significant after adjusting for patient preference for TJR (measured using a single item question). In the second study,[29] Hausmann et al. analyzed audio recordings for 402 of the 526 patients in the cohort to examine racial differences in patient-provider communication about treatment of chronic knee and hip osteoarthritis. The authors found very little racial difference in patient-provider communication, including no difference in informed decision-making and no difference in visit length, provider or patient affect, or physician verbal dominance. The only 2 aspects of communication that differed were less discussion of biomedical topics and more rapport-building statements in visits with blacks compared with whites. The authors conclude that their findings argue against the idea that communication differences play a large role in explaining disparities in joint replacement.

Finally, a small pilot study testing an intervention designed to reduce joint disparities in VA[44] contains data on baseline racial disparities. (The results of the intervention are described below.) The study included a convenience sample of 102 patients with moderate to severe osteoarthritis (WOMAC >39) recruited from the Greater Los Angeles VA Healthcare System. Baseline expectations about post-TKR outcome were lower for African American patients than for white patients regarding pain and physical function (P= 0.18 and P=0.13, respectively), although the results were not statistically significant. African American patients were also less likely to have ever heard of TKR compared with whites (49% vs. 72%, p=0.02), and less likely to know someone who had TKR (34% vs. 53%, p=0.05). There was no statistically significant difference in willingness to consider surgery at baseline (P=0.12).

Summary of Findings

Evidence about the patient-, provider-, and system- level factors that contribute to disparities in joint replacement surgery in the VA comes from a series of small studies recruiting patients from one or two VA medical centers. The studies find generally that black patients, compared with whites, have lower expectations about the effectiveness of joint replacement, less familiarity with the procedure, and may be more likely to view prayer and other techniques as useful for managing arthritis pain. There is some evidence that blacks may be less likely to be referred to specialists for joint replacement or to have TJR recommended by a specialist; however, some of these differences may be explained by patient preferences. One study examining communication between patients and orthopedic surgeons in the VA found little difference by race.

Although the individual studies are of high quality, the overall quality of evidence for the above conclusions is low because the studies were small and limited to a few sites. It is also likely that further research into important mediators (such as patient preference) and research with different patient cohorts will have an important impact on conclusions about the reasons for these joint disparities. The age of the data is also a limiting factor: a majority of the studies come from patient cohorts recruited over 10 years ago, and 8 of those studies come from a single VA medical center.

Data about reasons for disparities for other races (Hispanic, Asian) are scant, and no conclusions can be drawn. The quality of evidence is therefore very low.

Non-VA Data

A number of review articles have been published about reasons for disparities in health care in general and a few about osteoarthritis and pain in particular. Perhaps most notable is the Institute of Medicine report "Unequal Treatment: Confronting Racial and Ethnic Disparities in Health Care."[63] This report concluded, with respect to "Assessing Potential Sources of Disparities in Care," that:

- A small number of studies suggest that racial and ethnic minority patients are more likely than white patients to refuse care. These studies find the differences in refusal rates are generally small and that minority patient refusal does not fully explain health care disparities.

- Many sources, including health systems, healthcare providers, patients, and utilization managers - may contribute to racial and ethnic disparities in healthcare.

- Bias, stereotyping, prejudice, and clinical uncertainty on the part of healthcare providers may contribute to racial and ethnic disparities in healthcare. While indirect evidence from several lines of research support this statement, a greater understanding of the prevalence and influence of these processes is needed and should be sought through research.

More recent review articles on disparities in general include that of King et al.,[64] which expanded somewhat on the IOM review, and Klonoff,[65] which noted that "almost 35% of the national differences in arthroplasty rates for African-American women and almost 95% of the differences for Latino women appear to reflect that African-American and Latino women were more likely to live in areas of the country with lower rates of arthroplasty". Saha et al.[66] reviewed disparities in VA health care and categorized potential causes of disparities as patient medical knowledge and information sources, patient trust and skepticism, patient participation, patient social support and resources, clinician judgment, racial/cultural milieu, and healthcare facility characteristics.

Reviews more specific to joint replacement include a section of a review by Anderson, Green and Payne[67] on disparities in pain, which concluded that variability in decision-making in primary care as well as delay in surgical referral contributed to disparities in pain and post-operative outcomes; and a review by Allen[68] on racial and ethnic disparities in osteoarthritis phenotypes, which concluded that knee osteoarthritis may be more common in African-Americans than in Caucasians in the United States, and that pain and problems with physical functioning is greater for African-Americans than for Caucasians with knee osteoarthritis.

Set against this general background, we identified 20 studies of non-VA disparities in joint replacement surgery that we classified as second-generation studies. Of these, four were also included in the review by Kane and colleagues.[69-72] These studies focused on a handful of topics including severity of OA, knowledge of joint replacement, perceived benefits and fear of surgery, consideration of surgery in the past, impact of socioeconomic factors, patient attitudes and beliefs, willingness-to-pay, referral to a surgeon, and receipt of surgery at a low volume hospital or by a low volume surgeon. An individual study could report on one or more of these topics.

Eight studies looked at knowledge, perceived benefits, or fear of joint replacement surgery.[57, 69-75] Three studies assessing knowledge of or familiarity with joint replacement surgery found that, in general, African-Americans had less knowledge than whites or were less likely to have known someone who had undergone this surgery.[69, 72, 75] African-Americans had greater fear before and after hip or knee arthroplasty than whites.[74] Another study found that health beliefs differed by race/ethnicity. Trust was a critical issue for Hispanic patients, while overall economic issues were less important.[74]

In race-based focus groups, Whites, Hispanics, and African-Americans differed in their explanations of causal factors for OA, the change in lifestyle from OA, their trust of and skepticism about the physician, and payment for TKR.[76] African-Americans reported low expectations that TKR would improve their joint pain or health,[70] but there was no comparison race/ethnicity group in this particular study. Expectations about joint replacement surgery were lower among African-American men relative to white women, even after adjustment of socioeconomic factors.[57] Whites were more likely to consider TKR surgery beneficial.[69] One study using race concordant facilitators for focus groups suggested that differences in health beliefs and attitudes about surgery were primarily based on personal experiences; contrary to the other studies, the study concluded that African-Americans did not have more concerns/fears or worse expectations than whites.[73] Another study's qualitative interviews with black participants reinforce the findings that blacks had a preference for natural remedies, negative expectations of surgery, beliefs about God's control, a preference for continuing in their current state, poor relationships with specialists, and fear of surgery or death.[71] One of the above studies did not find differences in self-treatment for joint pain.[75]

Four studies assessed aspects of pre-operative and/or post-operative function across different racial groups.[77-80] Two studies, one conducted at New York University hospital and another at University of Pennsylvania hospital, found that African Americans had worse pre-operative knee function compared with whites, and longer delays to presentation for surgery. African American women had worse post-operative function, but the incremental gain with joint replacement surgery was equivalent to whites. Both studies support the hypothesis that African American patients present for TKR in a more advanced state than whites, but that improvement in function is approximately equivalent.

A third study examined the variation in family structure and social support between various racial groups after an individual had undergone hip fracture surgery or lower extremity joint replacement. The study found that whites and blacks were statistically significantly more likely to be responsible for their own care and discharged home alone than were Hispanics or Asians.[79] These differences in family structure and social support appear to be related to outcome disparities, with Hispanic males being the least likely to report hospital readmission at follow-up. Similarly, the last study found that blacks and Hispanics were more likely to be discharged to home following hip replacement, with Hispanics showing a statistically significant difference.[80] Men also had higher odds of being discharged to home. However, mean functional status change did not predict discharge disposition, suggesting that ethnic and gender disparities exist in THR care outcomes.

Three studies using administrative data (California State and New York City) found race/ethnic disparities for receipt of joint replacement surgery by a low volume hospital or low volume surgeon.[81, 82] Liu[82] found that African-Americans, Hispanics and Asians were more likely to receive TKR in low volume hospitals, controlling for socioeconomic factors, comorbidities and distance to hospital. SooHoo[83] also found that minorities as compared to white patients were more likely to undergo THR in low volume hospitals. Using New York City data, Epstein found that African-Americans, Hispanics, and Asians were more likely to receive total hip replacement in either a low volume hospital or by a low volume surgeon, also controlling for socioeconomic factors and distance to hospital.[81] These studies may support the hypothesis that "geography is destiny," meaning that where patients seek care largely influences the kinds and amount of care they receive.

Willingness-to-pay methodology was used in two studies by the same author group (both included the same subset of patients for the random dialing component). They found that African-Americans had a lower willingness-to-pay for TKR than whites,[84, 85] but differences were not significant in one study for Hispanics after adjusting for confounders.[85]

One study found that African-Americans patients were less likely to have seen an orthopedic surgeon for hip/knee surgery.[75] Physicians were more likely to discuss TKR with minorities (African-Americans and Hispanics), but whites were more likely to consider having surgery.[69] Ethnic differences remained after controlling for disease severity. African-Americans patients, especially women, had longer delays to getting TKR surgery.[77]

An old study (data from 1970s and 1980s) documents lower use of TKR among blacks compared with whites, even in the Medicaid-eligible or Medicare population, questioning whether economic factors alone explain the differences.[11] Another more recent study using data from the Health and Retirement Survey from 1998-2004 also found that relative poverty or access to care did not explain disparities between blacks and whites in receipt of joint replacement.[62]

Overall these studies are of moderate quality, and the results across studies and procedures are relatively consistent. We found few studies on Hispanics and Asians, and as such the evidence is of low quality for them.

Summary of Findings

Evidence in non-VA settings suggests that minority patients (African Americans being the most studied) may have less knowledge about joint replacement surgery, perceive fewer health benefits, and have greater fear about the surgery, similar to findings within VA. These patients may be less likely to be referred to a surgeon and are less likely to consider surgery. When they do present for surgery, African Americans have more advanced disease. Disease severity, socioeconomic factors, or degree of comorbidities do not appear to account for all of these differences. Minority patients may be less likely to be treated in high volume centers or by high volume providers, which is a system-level factor that has not been studied within VA.

KEY QUESTION #3. What is the evidence regarding VA or non-VA interventions to reduce disparities in joint replacement surgery?

We identified only one study of an intervention designed to reduce joint disparities in VA.[44] The authors assessed a decision aid that attempted to improve patient knowledge and expectations. The decision aid was a 45-minute videotape created by the Foundation for Informed Medical Decision Making about the treatment options for knee osteoarthritis, including total joint replacement. One hundred and two veterans from the Greater Los Angeles VA Healthcare System were recruited via flyers in VA clinics and waiting areas. Eligible subjects had to have moderate to severe osteoarthritis (as defined by the Western Ontario and McMaster Universities Osteoarthritis Index (WOMAC) of greater than 39) and have no significant medical comorbidities. Sixty-four subjects ended up watching the video, attending a focus group, and completing both pre- and post- video surveys about expectations regarding post-operative total knee replacement pain and function.

Compared with Caucasians, African Americans had worse pre-video expectations of pain and function following total knee replacement. After watching the video, expectations were unchanged for Caucasian veterans. However, African American veterans had statistically significant improvements in their expectations for pain and function post-operatively (see Table 3 below). The post-video expectations were therefore essentially the same for Caucasians and for African American veterans. The authors conclude that baseline disparities in expectations can be improved.

Table 3. Baseline and post-intervention total knee replacement expectations (n=64). Western Ontario and McMaster Universities Osteoarthritis Index (WOMAC) scale 0-100, where higher scores reflect poorer expectations.

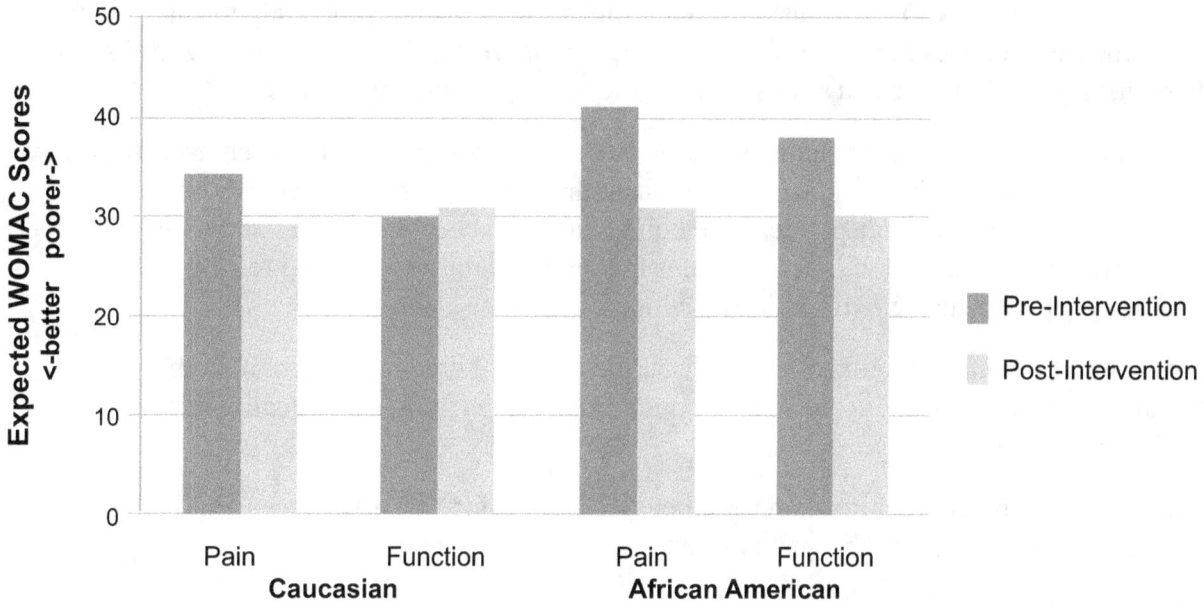

Summary of Findings

There has been only one published VA study of an intervention to improve disparities. It focused on expectations and examined only total knee replacement. Other potential causes of disparities have not been the subjects of interventions, and no study has yet assessed changes in the actual delivery of joint replacement surgery.

The quality of evidence for this key question is very low, due to sparseness of data; thus any estimate of effect is uncertain.

SUMMARY AND DISCUSSION

SUMMARY OF EVIDENCE BY KEY QUESTION

Key Question #1

What is the evidence about the existence and magnitude of disparities in joint replacement surgery in VA? How does this compare to published studies from non-VA US populations?

Data supporting existence of disparities in joint replacement surgery in VA are not very robust because they come from just three studies, two of which focus on racial disparities and one of which focuses on gender disparities. The magnitude of the racial disparities in VA as documented in these studies is about the same as the magnitude based on more extensive data from non-VA US populations (about 1.5-3 fold). The quality of evidence for this conclusion is low, based on sparseness and age of data. Thus we expect further research both into racial and gender disparities, to have an important impact on our estimate of the magnitude of disparities.

The literature on racial disparities in total joint replacement outside the VA is more robust than within the VA. Studies of non-VA US populations consistently find that black patients receive fewer TKR operations than whites, and men receive fewer TKR operations than women. The quality of evidence for this conclusion is high; thus future research is unlikely to change our confidence about the estimate of effect. However, future research is still necessary to evaluate these disparities over time and assess whether they are increasing or decreasing.

There are fewer studies that examine whether differences in TKR rates represent true disparities based on clinical need. Those that have examined this issue conclude in general, but not consistently, that there are disparities based on clinical need between blacks and nonblacks. The quality of evidence for this conclusion is moderate. Further research is likely to affect our confidence in the estimate of disparities and may change the estimate.

Data about differences in utilization and disparities for total hip replacement in both non-VA US and VA populations are scant, and no conclusions can be drawn. The quality of evidence is therefore very low.

Data about differences in utilization for other races (Hispanic, Asian) are scant, and no conclusions can be drawn. The quality of evidence is therefore very low.

Key Question #2

What is the evidence about the patient level, provider level, and system level factors that contribute to disparities in joint replacement surgery in VA? How does this compare to published studies from non-VA populations?

Only three studies combine both VA and non-VA patients and examine racial disparities in joint replacement, but they are not able to directly compare actual disparities across VA and non-VA sites. In these studies, there were no racial differences in clinical appropriateness for TJR or differences in perceived arthritis severity or susceptibility for worsening. African American patients were less likely than whites to perceive benefits of and more likely to recognize barriers to TJR. There was no difference in clinical appropriateness for patients at a county hospital compared with patients at a nearby VA. Studies found that County hospital patients were nearly 3-fold more likely to be referred to a surgeon compared with VA patients, but this association was not significant when self-reported referral data were used. The quality of evidence for this conclusion is low because all data came from a single cohort, and replication of the results in other patient populations is needed in order to have stronger confidence in the conclusion.

Evidence about the patient-, provider-, and system- level factors that contribute to disparities in joint replacement surgery in the VA comes from a series of small studies recruiting patients from one or two VA medical centers. The studies find generally that black patients, compared with whites, have lower expectations about the effectiveness of joint replacement, less familiarity with the procedure, and may be more likely to view prayer and other techniques as useful for managing arthritis pain. There is some evidence that blacks may be less likely to be referred to specialists for joint replacement or to have TJR recommended by a specialist; however, some of these differences may be explained by patient preferences. One study examining communication between patients and orthopedic surgeons in the VA found little difference by race.

Although the individual studies are of high quality, the overall quality of evidence for the above conclusions is low because the studies were small and limited to a few sites. It is also likely that further research into important mediators (such as patient preference) and research with different patient cohorts will have an important impact on conclusions about the reasons for these joint disparities. The age of the data is also a limiting factor: a majority of the studies come from patient cohorts recruited over 10 years ago, and 8 of those studies come from a single VA medical center.

Data about reasons for disparities for other races (Hispanic, Asian) are scant, and no conclusions can be drawn. The quality of evidence is therefore very low.

Evidence in non-VA settings suggests that minority patients (African Americans being the most studied) may have less knowledge about joint replacement surgery, perceive fewer health benefits, and have greater fear about the surgery, similar to findings within VA. These patients may be less likely to be referred to a surgeon and are less likely to consider surgery. When they do present for surgery, African Americans have more advanced disease. Disease severity, socioeconomic factors, or degree of comorbidities do not appear to account for all of these differences. Minority patients may be less likely to be treated in high volume centers or by high volume providers, which is a system-level factor that has not been studied within VA.

Key Question #3

What is the evidence regarding VA or non-VA interventions to reduce disparities in joint replacement surgery?

There has been only one published VA study of an intervention to improve disparities. It focused on expectations and examined only total knee replacement. It found that, after watching an informational video, African Americans, but not Caucasians, had statistically significant improvements in their expectations for pain and function post-operatively. Other potential causes of disparities have not been the subjects of interventions, and no study has yet assessed changes in the actual delivery of joint replacement surgery.

The quality of evidence for this key question is very low, due to sparseness of data; thus any estimate of effect is uncertain.

LIMITATIONS

Publication Bias

Our literature search procedures were extensive and included canvassing experts from academia regarding studies we may have missed. It was not possible to conduct formal tests for publication bias, but even with such tests it is not possible to exclude the possibility that such bias exists. Therefore, readers are cautioned about this possibility.

Study Quality

An important limitation common to systematic reviews is the quality of the original studies. We did not identify any randomized studies. For non-randomized studies, we adapted from the Newcastle Ottawa Scale those criteria most applicable to our purposes, namely items about the representativeness of the enrolled population, the potential for misclassification bias in the identification of race, gender, or receipt of procedure, and the response rate or follow-up rate. Several studies that used non-VA data were based on nationally representative populations. This was in general not the case for the VA studies, which tended to be from one or two institutions.

Types of Factors Evaluated

Almost all studies of factors potentially contributing to disparities were of patient or provider-level factors. System-level factors that are amenable to quality improvement activities, such as waiting times, have rarely been addressed.

Applicability of Findings to the VA Population

For the VA studies we assessed, the results are directly applicable to the VA population. However, as noted, the studies were generally restricted to only one or two centers.

Types of Disparities Represented in the Literature

While our search for disparities was broad, we identified a body of literature that deals primarily with disparities in race and gender. Other potential disparities, such as educational and socioeconomic factors, have been largely unstudied.

RECOMMENDATIONS FOR FUTURE RESEARCH

More research is needed in VA. The one national study of disparities in joint replacement in VA[27] contain data from over 10 years ago and focused on knee replacement only, and the second uses more recent data[26] but includes individuals referred to orthopedic clinics at two VA (with borderline statistical significance for the finding of racial disparities after statistical adjustment). Most VA second-generation studies are from limited samples and are over ten years old. The reviewed VA studies were well-designed, but a better and more current understanding of the reasons for the observed disparities is needed in order to design third-generation intervention studies that are most likely to succeed. In addition, with the increasing number of women and Hispanic veterans, planning now to better understand their potential need for TJR in the future is warranted.

In specific, VA could consider assessing the current utilization of TJR in a national or representative sample of veterans and VISNs, to first establish the magnitude of any differences in utilization in TJR between male and female veterans and those of different races. Second, presuming current data confirm the presence of different utilization rates, an in-depth examination should be performed of the degree to which these may be confounded by other factors, in other words asses "need" for joint replacement. Third, presuming that, even after adjusting for confounders, there still exists differential utilization among Veterans of different gender and ethnicity with the same "need," mixed-method types of research will be necessary to help establish the causes and barriers that are contributing to this disparity. This research should examine, in addition to patient and provider level factors, the kinds of system level factors that are particularly amenable to the types of quality improvement initiatives that VA can implement well, due to its organizational structure. Lastly, based on the results of all the above, VA should test interventions to diminish disparities, addressing the need for third generation work, and implement those found effective nationally.

REFERENCES

1. DuBard, C. A., et al., Racial/ethnic differences in quality of care for North Carolina Medicaid recipients. *N C Med J,* 2009. 70(2): p. 96-101.

2. Lillie-Blanton, M., et al., Race, ethnicity, and the health care system: public perceptions and experiences. *Med Care Res Rev,* 2000. 57 Suppl 1: p. 218-35.

3. Consensus development conference statement: total knee replacement. 2003, National Institute of Health.

4. Kane, R. L., et al., Total knee replacement. Evidence Report/Technology Assessment No. 86 (Prepared by the Minnesota Evidence-based Practice Center, Minneapolis, MN). in *AHRQ Publication.* 2003, Agency for Healthcare Research and Quality: Rockville, MD. No. 04-E006-2.

5. NIH consensus conference: total hip replacement. NIH consensus development panel on total hip replacement. *JAMA,* 1995. 273: p. 1950-1956.

6. Hochberg, M. C., et al., Guidelines for the medical management of osteoarthritis. Part II. Osteoarthritis of the knee. American College of Rheumatology. *Arthritis Rheum,* 1995. 38(11): p. 1541-6.

7. Dieppe, P., et al., Knee replacement surgery for osteoarthritis: effectiveness, practice variations, indications and possible determinants of utilization. *Rheumatology* (Oxford), 1999. 38(1): p. 73-83.

8. Escarce, J. J., et al., Racial differences in the elderly's use of medical procedures and diagnostic tests. *Am J Public Health,* 1993. 83(7): p. 948-54.

9. Baron, J. A., et al., Total hip arthroplasty: use and select complications in the US Medicare population. *Am J Public Health,* 1996. 86(1): p. 70-2.

10. Sharkness, C. M., et al., Prevalence of artificial hip implants and use of health services by recipients. *Public Health Rep,* 1993. 108(1): p. 70-5.

11. Wilson, M. G., D. S. May and J. J. Kelly, Racial differences in the use of total knee arthroplasty for osteoarthritis among older Americans. *Ethn Dis,* 1994. 4(1): p. 57-67.

12. Hoaglund, F. T., C. S. Oishi and G. G. Gialamas, Extreme variations in racial rates of total hip arthroplasty for primary coxarthrosis: a population-based study in San Francisco. *Ann Rheum Dis,* 1995. 54(2): p. 107-10.

13. Katz, J. N., et al., Can comorbidity be measured by questionnaire rather than medical record review? *Med Care,* 1996. 34(1): p. 73-84.

14. Giacomini, M. K., Gender and ethnic differences in hospital-based procedure utilization in California. *Arch Intern Med,* 1996. 156(11): p. 1217-24.

15.   Escalante, A., et al., Recipients of hip replacement for arthritis are less likely to be His-
       panic, independent of access to health care and socioeconomic status. *Arthritis Rheum,*
       2000. 43(2): p. 390-9.

16.   Mehrotra, C., et al., Trends in total knee replacement surgeries and implications for pub-
       lic health, 1990-2000. *Public Health Rep,* 2005. 120(3): p. 278-82.

17.   Ibrahim, S. A., Racial variations in the utilization of knee and hip joint replacement: an
       introduction and review of the most recent literature. *Curr Orthop Pract.* 21(2): p. 126-
       131.

18.   Morgan, R. C., Jr. and J. Slover, Breakout session: Ethnic and racial disparities in joint
       arthroplasty. *Clin Orthop Relat Res.* 469(7): p. 1886-90.

19.   Singh, J. A., Epidemiology of knee and hip arthroplasty: a systematic review. *Open Or-
       thop J.* 5: p. 80-5.

20.   Kane, R. L., et al., Disparities in total knee replacements: a review. *Arthritis Rheum,*
       2007. 57(4): p. 562-7.

21.   Wennberg, J. E., The geography of health care in the United States, in *The Dartmouth
       atlas of health care,* J. E. Wennberg and C. M. McAndrew, Editors. 1996, American Pub-
       lishing, Inc.: Chicago. p. 11-35.

22.   Wennberg, J. E., Dealing with medical practice variations: a proposal for action. *Health
       Aff* (Millwood), 1984. 3(2): p. 6-32.

23.   Jadad, A. R., et al., Assessing the quality of reports of randomized clinical trials: is blind-
       ing necessary? *Control Clin Trials,* 1996. 17(1): p. 1-12.

24.   Wells, G., et al. The Newcastle-Ottawa Scale (NOS) for assessing the quality of nonran-
       domised studies in meta-analyses 2000; Available from: http://www.ohri.ca/programs/
       clinical_epidemiology/oxford.asp.

25.   Kilbourne, A. M., et al., Advancing health disparities research within the health care sys-
       tem: a conceptual framework. *Am J Public Health,* 2006. 96(12): p. 2113-21.

26.   Hausmann, L. R., et al., The Effect of Patient Race on Total Joint Replacement Recom-
       mendations and Utilization in the Orthopedic Setting. *J Gen Intern Med,* 2010.

27.   Jones, A., et al., Racial disparity in knee arthroplasty utilization in the veterans health
       administration. *Arthritis Rheum,* 2005. 53(6): p. 979-81.

28.   Ibrahim, S. A., et al., Racial/ethnic differences in surgical outcomes in veterans following
       knee or hip arthroplasty. *Arthritis Rheum,* 2005. 52(10): p. 3143-51.

29.   Hausmann, L. R., et al., Orthopedic communication about osteoarthritis treatment: does
       patient race matter? *Arthritis Care Res,* 2011. 63(5): p. 635-642.

30.   Ang, D. C., G. James and T. E. Stump, Clinical appropriateness and not race predicted
       referral for joint arthroplasty. *Arthritis Rheum,* 2009. 61(12): p. 1677-85.

31. Ang, D. C., et al., African Americans and Whites are equally appropriate to be considered for total joint arthroplasty. *J Rheumatol,* 2009. 36(9): p. 1971-6.

32. Ang, D. C., P. O. Monahan and T. A. Cronan, Understanding ethnic disparities in the use of total joint arthroplasty: application of the health belief model. *Arthritis Rheum,* 2008. 59(1): p. 102-8.

33. Jones, A. C., et al., Investigating racial differences in coping with chronic osteoarthritis pain. *J Cross Cult Gerontol,* 2008. 23(4): p. 339-47.

34. Groeneveld, P. W., et al., Racial differences in expectations of joint replacement surgery outcomes. *Arthritis Rheum,* 2008. 59(5): p. 730-7.

35. Weng, H. H. and J. Fitzgerald, Current issues in joint replacement surgery. *Curr Opin Rheumatol,* 2006. 18(2): p. 163-9.

36. Lopez, J. P., et al., Patient perceptions of access to care and referrals to specialists: a comparison of African-American and white older patients with knee and hip osteoarthritis. *J Natl Med Assoc,* 2005. 97(5): p. 667-73.

37. Ang, D. C., et al., Is there a difference in the perception of symptoms between african americans and whites with osteoarthritis? *J Rheumatol,* 2003. 30(6): p. 1305-10.

38. Ibrahim, S. A., et al., Older patients' perceptions of quality of chronic knee or hip pain: differences by ethnicity and relationship to clinical variables. *J Gerontol A Biol Sci Med Sci,* 2003. 58(5): p. M472-7.

39. Ibrahim, S. A., et al., Differences in expectations of outcome mediate African American/ white patient differences in "willingness" to consider joint replacement. *Arthritis Rheum,* 2002. 46(9): p. 2429-35.

40. Ang, D. C., et al., Ethnic differences in the perception of prayer and consideration of joint arthroplasty. *Med Care,* 2002. 40(6): p. 471-6.

41. Ibrahim, S. A., et al., Self-assessed global quality of life: a comparison between African-American and white older patients with arthritis. *J Clin Epidemiol,* 2002. 55(5): p. 512-7.

42. Ibrahim, S. A., et al., Understanding ethnic differences in the utilization of joint replacement for osteoarthritis: the role of patient-level factors. *Med Care,* 2002. 40(1 Suppl): p. I44-51.

43. Ibrahim, S. A., et al., Variation in perceptions of treatment and self-care practices in elderly with osteoarthritis: a comparison between African American and white patients. *Arthritis Rheum,* 2001. 45(4): p. 340-5.

44. Weng, H. H., et al., Development of a decision aid to address racial disparities in utilization of knee replacement surgery. *Arthritis Rheum,* 2007. 57(4): p. 568-75.

45. Borrero, S., et al., Brief report: Gender and total knee/hip arthroplasty utilization rate in the VA system. *J Gen Intern Med,* 2006. 21 Suppl 3: p. S54-7.

46.   Hawker, G. A., et al., Differences between men and women in the rate of use of hip and knee arthroplasty. *N Engl J Med,* 2000. 342(14): p. 1016-22.

47.   Skinner, J., et al., Racial, ethnic, and geographic disparities in rates of knee arthroplasty among Medicare patients. *N Engl J Med,* 2003. 349(14): p. 1350-9.

48.   Escalante, A., et al., Disparity in total hip replacement affecting Hispanic Medicare beneficiaries. *Med Care,* 2002. 40(6): p. 451-60.

49.   Katz, B. P., et al., Demographic variation in the rate of knee replacement: a multi-year analysis. *Health Serv Res,* 1996. 31(2): p. 125-40.

50.   McBean, A. M. and M. Gornick, Differences by race in the rates of procedures performed in hospitals for Medicare beneficiaries. *Health Care Financ Rev,* 1994. 15(4): p. 77-90.

51.   Racial disparities in total knee replacement among Medicare enrollees--United States, 2000-2006. *MMWR Morb Mortal Wkly Rep,* 2009. 58(6): p. 133-8.

52.   Jha, A. K., et al., Racial trends in the use of major procedures among the elderly. *N Engl J Med,* 2005. 353(7): p. 683-91.

53.   Skinner, J., W. Zhou and J. Weinstein, The influence of income and race on total knee arthroplasty in the United States. *J Bone Joint Surg Am,* 2006. 88(10): p. 2159-66.

54.   Hawkins, K., et al., Disparities in Major Joint Replacement Surgery among Adults with Medicare Supplement Insurance. *Popul Health Manag.*

55.   Jain, N. B., et al., Trends in epidemiology of knee arthroplasty in the United States, 1990-2000. *Arthritis Rheum,* 2005. 52(12): p. 3928-33.

56.   Bang, H., et al., Total hip and total knee arthroplasties: trends and disparities revisited. *Am J Orthop* (Belle Mead NJ). 39(9): p. E95-102.

57.   Hanchate, A. D., et al., Exploring the determinants of racial and ethnic disparities in total knee arthroplasty: health insurance, income, and assets. *Med Care,* 2008. 46(5): p. 481-8.

58.   Olson, J. C. and J. Foland, Tracking racial and ethnic disparities of knee replacement rates in Connecticut. *Conn Med,* 2005. 69(4): p. 211-5.

59.   Basu, J. and L. R. Mobley, Trends in racial disparities among the elderly for selected procedures. *Med Care Res Rev,* 2008. 65(5): p. 617-37.

60.   Oishi, C. S., et al., Total hip replacement rates are higher among Caucasians than Asians in Hawaii. Clin Orthop Relat Res, 1998(353): p. 166-74.

61.   Francis, M. L., et al., Joint replacement surgeries among medicare beneficiaries in rural compared with urban areas. *Arthritis Rheum,* 2009. 60(12): p. 3554-62.

62.   Steel, N., et al., Racial disparities in receipt of hip and knee joint replacements are not explained by need: the Health and Retirement Study 1998-2004. *J Gerontol A Biol Sci Med Sci,* 2008. 63(6): p. 629-34.

63.   Unequal Treament: Confronting Racial and Ethnic Disparities in Health Care. Institute of Medicine, ed. B. D. Smedley, A. Y. Stith and A. R. Nelson. 2002, Washington, DC: National Academy Press.

64.   King, R. K., et al., A plan for action: key perspectives from the racial/ethnic disparities strategy forum. *Milbank Q,* 2008. 86(2): p. 241-72.

65.   Klonoff, E. A., Disparities in the provision of medical care: an outcome in search of an explanation. *J Behav Med,* 2009. 32(1): p. 48-63.

66.   Saha, S., et al., Racial and ethnic disparities in the VA health care system: a systematic review. *J Gen Intern Med,* 2008. 23(5): p. 654-71.

67.   Anderson, K. O., C. R. Green and R. Payne, Racial and ethnic disparities in pain: causes and consequences of unequal care. *J Pain,* 2009. 10(12): p. 1187-204.

68.   Allen, K. D., Racial and ethnic disparities in osteoarthritis phenotypes. *Curr Opin Rheumatol.* 22(5): p. 528-32.

69.   Suarez-Almazor, M. E., et al., Ethnic variation in knee replacement: patient preferences or uninformed disparity? *Arch Intern Med,* 2005. 165(10): p. 1117-24.

70.   Figaro, M. K., P. Williams-Russo and J. P. Allegrante, Expectation and outlook: the impact of patient preference on arthritis care among African Americans. *J Ambul Care Manage,* 2005. 28(1): p. 41-8.

71.   Figaro, M. K., P. W. Russo and J. P. Allegrante, Preferences for arthritis care among urban African Americans: "I don't want to be cut". *Health Psychol,* 2004. 23(3): p. 324-9.

72.   Chang, H. J., et al., Concerns of patients actively contemplating total knee replacement: differences by race and gender. *Arthritis Rheum,* 2004. 51(1): p. 117-23.

73.   Suarez-Almazor, M. E., et al., A qualitative analysis of decision-making for total knee replacement in patients with osteoarthritis. *J Clin Rheumatol,* 2010. 16(4): p. 158-63.

74.   Lavernia, C. J., J. C. Alcerro and M. D. Rossi, Fear in arthroplasty surgery: the role of race. *Clin Orthop Relat Res,* 2010. 468(2): p. 547-54.

75.   Blake, V. A., et al., Racial differences in social network experience and perceptions of benefit of arthritis treatments among New York City Medicare beneficiaries with self-reported hip and knee pain. *Arthritis Rheum,* 2002. 47(4): p. 366-71.

76.   Kroll, T. L., et al., "Keep on truckin'" or "It's got you in this little vacuum": race-based perceptions in decision-making for total knee arthroplasty. *J Rheumatol,* 2007. 34(5): p. 1069-75.

77.   Kamath, A. F., et al., Ethnic and Gender Differences in the Functional Disparities after Primary Total Knee Arthroplasty. *Clin Orthop Relat Res,* 2010.

78. Slover, J. D., M. G. Walsh and J. D. Zuckerman, Sex and race characteristics in patients undergoing hip and knee arthroplasty in an urban setting. *J Arthroplasty,* 2010. 25(4): p. 576-80.

79. Ottenbacher, K. J., et al., Disparity in health services and outcomes for persons with hip fracture and lower extremity joint replacement. *Med Care,* 2003. 41(2): p. 232-41.

80. Berges, I. M., et al., Gender and ethnic differences in rehabilitation outcomes after hip-replacement surgery. *Am J Phys Med Rehabil,* 2008. 87(7): p. 567-72.

81. Epstein, A. J., B. H. Gray and M. Schlesinger, Racial and ethnic differences in the use of high-volume hospitals and surgeons. *Arch Surg,* 2010. 145(2): p. 179-86.

82. Liu, J. H., et al., Disparities in the utilization of high-volume hospitals for complex surgery. *JAMA,* 2006. 296(16): p. 1973-80.

83. SooHoo, N. F., E. Farng and D. S. Zingmond, Disparities in the utilization of high-volume hospitals for total hip replacement. *J Natl Med Assoc.* 103(1): p. 31-5.

84. Byrne, M. M., et al., Racial/ethnic differences in preferences for total knee replacement surgery. *J Clin Epidemiol,* 2006. 59(10): p. 1078-86.

85. Byrne, M. M., K. J. O'Malley and M. E. Suarez-Almazor, Ethnic differences in health preferences: analysis using willingness-to-pay. *J Rheumatol,* 2004. 31(9): p. 1811-8.

APPENDIX A. SEARCH STRATEGY

 LIBRARY

HIP & KNEE REPLACEMENT – DISPARITIES

DATABASE SEARCHED:
 PubMed

TIME PERIOD COVERED: 1966-2010

LANGUAGE:
 ENGLISH

SEARCH STRATEGY:
arthroplasty, replacement, hip OR arthroplasty, replacement, knee OR arthritis/surgery OR osteoarthritis, knee/surgery OR osteoarthritis, hip/surgery OR (hip AND surger*(OR (knee AND surger*) OR (joint AND replac*) OR (knee AND replac*) OR (hip AND replac*) OR (joint AND arthroplast*) OR (hip AND arthroplast*) OR (knee AND arthroplast*)

AND
minority groups OR african americans OR hispanic americans OR african continental ancestry group OR racial OR ethnic OR minorities OR gender OR sex OR age[ti] OR age distribution

AND
disparity OR disparities OR difference* OR variation*

APPENDIX B. STUDY SELECTION FORM

Article ID:	**Reviewer:**
Authors:	
Title:	

1. What type of joint replacement is discussed? (Check all that apply)

   Total Knee Replacement (TKR) ....☐
   Total Hip Replacement (THR)...............☐
   Other: (specify_____) ...☐
   None..☐
   If None→ Stop

2. What type of disparity is discussed? (Check all that apply)

   Racial/ethnic...☐
   Gender...☐
   Urban/rural..☐
   Regional ....☐
   Socioeconomic status..............................☐
   Other: (specify_____) ...☐
   Not clear, needs further review ....☐
   None...☐
   If None→ Stop

3. Which generation of study does this best fit? (See explanation below for reference)
   First ....☐
   Second...☐
   Third..☐

5. Are veterans discussed, either as the main focus or as a sub-category?
   Main focus...☐
   Sub-category ....☐
   No mention...☐

6. What is the study design?
   Descriptive/observational.......................☐
   Experimental ....☐
   Qualitative...☐
   Systematic review or Meta-Analysis ......☐
   Other...☐

7. What is the approximate sample size?
   <100 ....☐
   100-500 ....☐
   >500 ....☐

8. Study origin?
   Unclear...☐
   US...☐
   Non-US ....☐
       Specify: _____

9. Mark as Background Article ....☐

- **First-Generation** studies document the *existence and the magnitude* of the disparities.
- **Second-generation** studies examine the *reasons for observed disparities* and could be classified as: a) patient-level factors (treatment preferences, patterns of self-care, etc.); b) provider-level factors (physician-patient communication, etc.); and c) system level factors (access to specialist care, etc.).
- **Third-generation** studies examine *interventions* to address the observed disparities.

APPENDIX C. DATA EXTRACTION FORM

ID: Reviewer:
Author:
Title:

1. Is the study based solely in the US?

   Yes..☐

   No.. ☐ STOP

2. Does the article examine an intervention to address the

   Yes..☐

   If Yes, specify:_____

   No..☐

3. What is the data source for the study? (check all that apply)

   a. Single institution ....☐

   b. Multi-institutional (Regional) ....☐

   c. Multi-institutional (National) ....☐

   d. VA (single or multi-VA) ....☐

   e. Medicare ....☐

   f. Medicaid ....☐

   g. NIS ....☐

   h. Other (Specify:_____)................☐

4. Who are the primary study subjects? (check all)

   a. Patients ....☐

   b. Providers..☐

   c. Other ....☐

5. How were patients selected?

   a. Population-based/systematic/representative .. sample… ....☐

   b. Consecutive patients..................................☐

   c. Convenience/non-representative sample ....☐

   d. Combination of above ....☐

   e. Unclear/unknown ....☐

6. Years of data collection covered*: _____

7. What is the study design?

   a. Cross-sectional… ....☐

   b. Cohort/Case-control ....☐

   c. Experimental ....☐

   d. Systematic Review....................................☐

   e. Unclear/unknown ....☐

   f. Background .... ☐STOP

8. What is/are the Primary Outcome Measure(s)?

   a. Receipt of procedure(s)..............................☐

   b. Recommendation for procedure(s) ....☐

   c. Outcome of Procedure ....☐

   d. Appropriateness for Procedure ....☐

   e. Perception of Need for Surgery ....☐

   f. Willingness to Consider Surgery ....☐

   g. Outcome Expectations of Surgery ....☐

   h. Other ....☐

      Specify: _____

      Specify: _____

9. What is/are the Secondary Outcome Measure(s)?

   a. Receipt of procedure(s)..............................☐

   b. Recommendation For procedure(s)..........☐

   c. Outcome of Procedure ....☐

   d. Appropriateness for Procedure ....☐

   e. Perception of Need for Surgery ....☐

   f. Willingness to Consider Surgery..............☐

   g. Outcome Expectations of Surgery ....☐

   h. Not Applicable ....☐

   i. Other..☐

      Specify: _____

      Specify: _____

      Specify: _____

10. **For Race:** How was race categorized?

    a. White .... ☐

    b. Black .... ☐

    c. Hispanic .... ☐

    d. Asian .... ☐

    e. Non-black .... ☐

    f. Non-white .... ☐

    g. None .... ☐

11. **For Race:** How was race determined?

    a. Administrative data .... ☐

    b. Medical record review .... ☐

    c. Self-reported .... ☐

    d. Two or more sources .... ☐

    e. Unknown or not reported .... ☐

12. Assessment of receipt of procedure

    a. Medical record .... ☐

    b. Administrative data .... ☐

    c. Self report .... ☐

    d. Not reported/unknown .... ☐

    e. Not applicable .... ☐

13. Assessment of primary disparity outcome (function, quality of life, receipt of procedure, etc)

    a. Medical record .... ☐

    b. Administrative data .... ☐

    c. Self report .... ☐

    d. Not reported/unknown .... ☐

14. Population sample size:

    a. Total_____

    b. Veteran sample size _____

15. What was the mean/median age of the patients*?

    _____

16. Response Rate

    a. Number Eligible for Study

    _____

    b. Number Declining Participation

    _____

    c. Response Rate if Reported_____

    d. Unclear/unspecified .... ☐

    e. Not applicable .... ☐

17. Adequacy of follow-up for subjects?

    a. Complete follow-up of all subjects .... ☐

    b. Subjects lost to follow-up .... ☐

       If so, # _____ or % _____ f/u

    c. Description of those lost to f/u .... ☐

    d. Unclear/unspecified .... ☐

    e. Not applicable .... ☐

18. If results were adjusted, were the following covariates included?

    a. Age .... ☐

    b. Gender .... ☐

    c. Income .... ☐

    d. Education .... ☐

    e. Insurance .... ☐

    f. Not Applicable .... ☐

19. **For Race**: How many "unknowns" were reported?

    a. Total or percent "unknown" .... _____

    b. Not reported .... ☐

*No data denoted as 999

APPENDIX D. Newcastle Ottawa Scale Criteria Used in Quality Assessment

Selection

1) Representativeness of the exposed cohort
2) Ascertainment of exposure
3) Demonstration that outcome of interest was not present at start of study

Comparability

1) Comparability of cohorts on the basis of the design or analysis

Outcome

1) Assessment of outcome
2) Was follow-up long enough for outcomes to occur
3) Adequacy of follow up of cohorts

APPENDIX E. PEER REVIEW COMMENTS/AUTHOR RESPONSES

Comment	Response
General Comments	
Issues such as waiting time, access to orthopedics consultations, etc. have not been clearly documented, and it is unknown if they may relate to some of the differences observed. If these barriers indeed exist, they should be addressed through quality improvement measures.	There is a new section in the limitations that addresses this.
Abbreviations not used consistently	After double-checking for inconsistencies, some remain due to the literature itself.
Missing: Hausmann, et al, Arthritis Care & Rheum 2011, p635-642	Now included, found in update search
In general the 'summary of findings' sections read better than the 'data' sections. The data sections need revision. Revisions to the data sections should be directed at reading fluency to better convey the intended message. Substantial editorial attention to writing, paragraph structure, style, grammar, and typographical errors is suggested.	Edits have been made to address this issue.
Authors may want to do a brief re-search, using the same database and keywords, for the period from January through June 2011 as a final update prior to publication.	Update is now included
I have some reservations about the level of evidence available to make any decisions of consequence. Although there is no documentation of the levels, it appears that most cited studies are at minimum a level III or IV. It would be helpful to document by the standard definitions and the numerical system to be sure everyone is on the same page. In addition, grades of recommendation for the consensus should use a standard nomenclature such as A,B,C,I, again for clarity. When levels of evidence are so low or the mass of supporting evidence is so low and recommendation can only be I, the only conclusion would be we need focused research of the highest quality and nothing more. In this current context, the supposed disparity may have no other basis than personal preference, cultural beliefs and population bias which may not be alterable.	The ESP program uses the GRADE system, which does not use the level I, II, III approach. The limitations of the evidence are reflected in the overall "quality of evidence," and most of these are rated as low or very low.
Executive Summary	
The summary was a little vague with respect to results. Since many individuals may only access the summary, a more precise summary of results would be appropriate, such as including how many studies were available for each key question, and whether they included or not VA populations. In general, the findings are reported as 'few studies...' or 'most....'. Including number of studies and participants would be useful. This is all included in the main report, but would be useful in the summary.	We have revised the executive summary to include more detail
2nd paragraphs notes there are "disparities" in TJR use in non-VA settings. It would be useful here to mention types of disparities that are being alluded to (e.g., race, gender, ethnicity...)	This paragraph has been updated to be more specific.
page 2, Key Question #1, 2nd paragraph notes that future research is unlikely to change confidence on the estimate of the effect. It should be qualified here (and elsewhere in the synthesis where this is also mentioned) that future research is still important for evaluating whether there are any temporal trends in disparities (e.g., do these change over time in response to any policies, interventions, etc).	Very good point, we have updated the relevant sections accordingly.

A Comparison of Joint Replacement Disparities in VA and Non-VA Settings: A Systematic Review

Comment	Response
On page 2 in the executive summary—it would be nice in the summary to add the number of studies contributing to the literature for each KQ	These numbers have been added at the beginning of the results section.
Background	
In the Background on page 1, page 5, and elsewhere the report refers to "disparities." This description is too general because the report only addresses gender and racial disparities. Clarification of this usage to use language such as "gender and racial disparities" in place of "disparities" is suggested.	We revised the draft to clarify.
The authors are limited by research papers which primarily address only two racial / ethnic groups (White, and African-American) and don't clearly address educational, socioeconomic and regional effects.	This is a limitation of the primary literature. Almost all the disparity literature deals with gender and race. Even within gender disparities, VA data are very scarce. These additional potential sources of disparities are now noted in the limitations.
Methods	
Search strategy includes 'peer-reviewed' articles. How is this assessed? Do the authors mean original publications? If reviews were included, how was it determined if they were peer-reviewed	We revised this to indicate that anything indexed on PubMed was potentially eligible
In the Methods (page 6) under the heading 'search strategy' more detailed description of the search terms should be provided. At a minimum indicate the surgical procedures THR and TKR.	We have added some of our specific terms, and the entire search strategy is in Appendix A.
Flow	
Figure 3 Literature Flow seems to have a discrepancy in the number of articles categorized in the bottom row of boxes. There are 22+35+1 = 58 studies categorized in the bottom row. The row above indicates there were 69 articles assessed. So it seems there are 11 articles (69 minus 58 = 11) that are not categorized.	Additional explanations have been added to clarify the overlapping nature of the categories, which accounts for the numerical discrepancy.
Figure 3 - It may also be useful to provide a breakdown of which or how many articles addressed racial disparities and how many addressed gender disparities. The current breakdown seems to indicate only 1 article addressed gender disparities	This is correct, there was only one gender article.
I can't follow Figure 3 and the numbers. It says 69 articles were assessed but the numbers below don't add up. Please clarify/fix. Also, I think it would help the reader to explain the literature groups below the figure.	Additional explanations have been added to clarify the overlapping nature of the categories, and the groups are now referred to by key question, rather than generation, for clarity.
Study Design	
Authors state that study design was not used as inclusion/exclusion criterion. However, Figure 3 includes inappropriate study design as a rejection criterion.	We have reworded the figure to be more specific.
Results	
The first set of results for Key Question #2 is related to a comparison of VA and non-VA county hospitals. It would be helpful to the reader if there is a clear statement about how these data relate to the key questions (e.g. differences according to a system-level factor?).	Updates have been made to address this.

Comment	Response
Page 12 – 2nd paragraph under VA Data, 3rd sentence – it is not completely clear what the comparison is for the OR, and there is a grammar issue in the sentence.	This sentence has been updated.
Page 12, three studies are alluded to – is the 2nd paragraph in this section about the third study?	Yes, this has been noted in the text.
Page 12, 2nd paragraph – which ICD-9 codes were used?	ICD-9 codes have been added where necessary
Page 13, 3rd paragraph under Non-VA data: some discussion of the magnitude of differences in TKR rates would be helpful.	The Kane review (published in arthritis care and research), does not list actual rates of use, just that rates in one group are larger or smaller than others. We think that the rates presented in the following studies below can present a sense of magnitude of differences in rates.
Page 17, Summary of Findings – doesn't fully summarize the results (or lack thereof) regarding patient, provider, and system level factors.	Changes have been made.
In some places it is clear which cohort is being referred to, in other places it is less clear (e.g., "another VA cohort" on p18, 2nd paragraph). Throughout, it would be helpful to have a consistent way of referring to each study in the table.	Updates have been made to better identify the cohort (e.g. the Cleveland cohort)
It is not clear that the general information under Non-VA Data that starts on p21 is needed. It seems a bit out of place here.	This section has been updated for better flow.
P24, Summary of findings – it would be helpful to compare / contrast this with VA data, mentioning any different findings or just areas in which there may be more data for non-VA vs. VA.	Updates have been made to address this.
For KQ1 there is one 'summary of findings' section at the end that includes both VA and non-VA data. For KQ2, the structure differs and was confusing at first – that is, within the KQ2 sections there are three 'summary' sections for each of VA + non-VA, VA, and non-VA.	This structure was used due to the volume of literature in the sections.
There is only one study examining gender disparities in the VA. This finding of limited research related to gender is not highlighted in the summary of findings.	The summary has been updated to reflect this.
Note: on page 12, first sentence under VA data––I think you want a "the" before VA. Also, in the 2nd paragraph, note there is a comma rather than a period in the pt estimate of 0.3 %	Changes have been made.
page 16––para 30–– fix tense of first sentence. Note also that the last sentence of this paragraph does not explain what the 2 fold higher odds are of????	This sentence has been removed.
Page 17. Please clarify last sentence of 2nd paragraph	Edits have been made to address this issue.
Page 18. 2nd paragraph, 2nd to last sentence–––I think you mean TJR rather than OA	OA has been verified.
Page 19-last sentence–––take out "thus"	Fixed
Page 23––-2nd paragraph––-review the middle sentence that states "social support between various racial groups after undergoing a hip fracture……	This sentence has been reworded for grammar and clarity.
It is hard to get too excited about KQ 3 since there seemed to be little good evidence about disparities in the VA. I might be clearer about the limitations of the VA data on disparities as you discuss an intervention to improve them in KQ3.	Noted

Comment	Response
Note also that in the first sentence the word "joint" probably doesn't belong there or you need to add TJR	Sentence has been verified.
Page 26 paragraph 4—since you are talking about the disparities, even if the data are not robust, I think you might as well say what you found in terms of the disparities. Also, I thought some of the differences were decreased with adjustment for confounders? This is a good place to reiterate that.	This is discussed in the "clinical need" paragraph. The differences may decrease after adjustment, but they don't go away entirely.
Page 27—KQ3. If you are going to talk about the one published study it makes sense to me to summarize what it showed	This has been added.
Recommendations for Future Research	
It would be appropriate to have more specific recommendations at the end of the review, arising from the evidence, or lack thereof. For instance: 1) areas with conflicting findings; 2) areas needed to be studied in Veterans, for which little information is available (e.g. women are mentioned, how about Hispanics); and 3) potential interventions that should be evaluated on the basis of the findings – patient-based or QI.	We have revised the future research section
This is a very comprehensive and detailed review of the literature, and it would be very helpful if more specific recommendations could be drafted in summary of the review. There may also be recommendations that could be made with respect to implementation, but given the current state of the research, it seems that more evidence base is needed regarding interventions to address disparities, before these are put into clinical practice. I think it will help readers / stakeholders to get more out of the evidence synthesis if a more detailed "take home" message is provided with respect to what is still needed.	We have revised the future research section
The report does not identify anything to implement. The call for more research seems appropriate	We have revised the future research section
I am not sure I agree with the recommendations for further research. it seems to me that if the evidence base is limited for first and second generation disparity studies that these should be conducted prior to suggesting more third generation research. it is not completely clear to me that there are disparities at the VA. I would like to see a Discussion section (it can be short) in this paper with some discussion of the problems with this evidence base. In particular, I am struck by how often point estimates of disparity were either reduced or eliminated by adjusting for confounders. I think this deserves more synthesis and discussion.	We have revised the future research section
Appendix F	
Appendix F. Number of articles is 57? The number does not match up with the numbers in Figure 3	Numbers have been updated.

APPENDIX F. EVIDENCE TABLES

Key Question 1/ Generation 1 Evidence Table

Author; Date	Data Dates*	Study Type; Sample Selection; Response Rate/ Follow Up	Total pop; VA pop*	Data Source	Gender, Race**/ How determined	Joint Discussed***	Outcomes	Results
VA Studies								
Hausmann; 2010[26]	2005-2008	Cohort/ Case-control; Unclear; Not specified	457; 457	VA, multi-institution	W/ Self-Reported	TKR, THR	recommendation for procedure; receipt of procedure	Lower odds of receiving a TJR recommendation for B than W of similar age and disease severity (OR 0.46, [95% CI 0.26–0.83]; P=0.01). Difference was not significant adjusting for patient preference for TJR (OR 0.69, [95% CI 0.36–1.31], P=0.25).TJR less likely for B than W of similar age and disease severity (OR 0.41 [95% CI 0.16–1.0], P=0.06); difference reduced adjusting for recommendation for procedure at the index visit (OR 0.57 [95% CI 0.21–1.54], P=0.27).
Borrero; 2006[45]	1999	Cross-sectional; Pop based; N/A	329,461; 329,461	VA National	Women/ Admin	TKR, THR	Adjusted odds of getting TJR	Among patients with OA, men and women in the VA were equally likely to undergo TKR (153 [1.6%] women and 4,638 [1.5%]) men and THR (73 [.8%] women and 2147 [.7%] men). Receipt of surgery within 2 years for women with OA versus men was not significant (TKR: OR 0.96 [95% CI 0.82 to 1.13]) and (THR: OR 0.99 [95% CI 0.79 to 1.26]).
Jones; 2005[27]	1999	Cohort/ Case-control; Pop based; Not specified	260856; 260856	VA National	W, B/ Admin. data	TKR	receipt of procedure	B were less likely than W to have received TKR within 2 years (OR 0.72, [95% CI 0.65–0.80] in OA cohort and OR 0.72, [95%CI 0.63–0.81] in specialty clinic subcohort.
Non-VA Studies								
Hawkins; 2011[54]	2006-2007	Cross-sectional; Pop-based; N/A	2.9 million; 0	Medigap	% non-white by zip code/ Admin	Hip or knee replacement	receipt of procedure	Patients living in high-minority areas were 20% less likely to undergo a hip or knee replacement as low minority areas.
Bang; 2010[56]	1996-2005	Cross-sectional; Pop-based; N/A	8000000	NIS	W, B, H, A/ Admin	TKR, THR	receipt of procedure	Non-whites had lower odds of THA and TKA compared with whites. Minorities were 23% to 64% less likely to undergo arthroplasties. Racial disparities were larger than income disparities and not confined to elderly or low-income.

43

Author; Date	Data Dates*	Study Type; Sample Selection; Response Rate/ Follow Up	Total pop; VA pop*	Data Source	Gender, Race**/ How determined	Joint Discussed***	Outcomes	Results
Francis; 2009[61]	2005	Cross-sectional; Pop-based; N/A	46000000; 0	Medicare, NIS	W, B, H, A/ Admin. data	TKR, THR	receipt of procedure	Compared with urban beneficiaries, rural were more likely to have TJR (OR 1.27 [95% CI 1.26–1.28]). Adjusting for age, sex, race/ethnicity, income, poverty ratio, and state, rural beneficiaries were still 14% more likely to have TJR (OR 1.14 [95% CI 1.13–1.16]).
2009[51]	2000/2006	Cross-sectional; Pop-based; N/A	26000000; N/A	Medicare	W, B/ Admin. data	TKR	receipt of procedure	From 2000 to 2006, TKR rate in the US increased 58%, from 5.5 to 8.7 per 1,000, with similar increases among W (61%) and B (56%). Rate of TKR for B was 37% lower than W in 2000 (3.6 versus 5.7 per 1,000) and 39% lower in 2006 (5.6 versus 9.2 per 1,000).
Basu; 2008[59]	1997-2001	Cross-sectional; Pop-based; N/A	71418; NR	National, HCUP	W, B, H/ Admin. data	THR	receipt of procedure	No difference in the likelihood of THR between B, W and H for 1997 or 2000, after adjusting for income, urban/rural, distance from hospital, and social isolation, but not severity of arthritis.
Steel; 2008[62]	1998, 2000, 2002	Cohort/ Case-control; Pop-based; Not specified	14807; NR	Health and retirement study, national	W, B/ Self-reported	TKR, THR	need for surgery; receipt of procedure	Lower receipt of TJR in B (vs W: OR 0.47; CI 0.26–0.83) or less educated (0.65; 0.44–0.96). Differences not explained by employment, access, family responsibilities, disability, living alone, comorbidity, or excluding younger than Medicare.
Hanchate; 2008[57]	1994-2004	Cohort/ Case-control; Pop-based; Not specified	18439; NR	National	W, B, H/ Self-reported	TKR	receipt of procedure	B men (relative to W women) were less likely (OR 0.46 (0.28–0.78), [P < 0.05]) to receive TKA. Adjusting for economic factors, racial/ethnicity, TKA rates differences for women disappeared, while remaining large for B men (OR 0.56 [0.33–0.95]).
Skinner; 2006[53]	2000 (Medi-care)	Cross-sectional; Pop-based; N/A	27494659; NR	NHANES, national Medicare	W, B, H, A/ Admin. data	TKR	receipt of procedure; Prevalence of OA	Relative to W men, B men were less likely to undergo TKA (OR 0.36 [95% CI 0.34 to 0.38); as were H men (OR 0.67 [0.62 to 0.73]; Asian men (OR 0.28 [0.24 to 0.32]; and Asian women (OR 0.45 [0.41 to 0.49]. W women were more likely (OR 1.34 [1.33 to 1.36]). [No income gradient for clinical and radiographic measures of arthritis, except a negative association of income and pain on passive motion (P<.05).]

Author; Date	Data Dates*	Study Type; Sample Selection; Response Rate/ Follow Up	Total pop; VA pop*	Data Source	Gender, Race**/ How determined	Joint Discussed***	Outcomes	Results
Jain; 2005[55]	1990-2000	Cross-sectional; Pop-based; N/A	443008; NR	NIS, national	W, B, H/ Admin. data	TKR	receipt of procedure	In 1998-2000 as compared to 1990-1993, B and Hispanic patients were more likely to undergo TKA (OR 1.6 [95% CI 1.5–1.6] and OR 2.7, [95% CI 2.5–2.9],respectively). However, W patients accounted for 87.5% and 93.0% of TKAs, in the 2 time periods.
Jha; 2005[52]	1992-2001	Cross-sectional; Pop-based; N/A	29000000; NR	Medicare	Non-B/ Admin. data	THR	receipt of procedure	Rates of TKR and THR among the Medicare fee for service population were compared from 1992 to 2001. Women had higher age-adjusted rates of procedure use than men, and nonblacks had higher rates than blacks. In 2001, nonblack men had a rate of 5.05/1000 population for TKR, compared to 1.85 for black men. Among women, rates of TKR per 1000 population were 6.6 among nonblacks and 5.1 among blacks.
Mehrotra; 2005[16]	1990-2000	Cross-sectional; Pop-based; N/A	67,475; NR	Regional (Wisconsin Hospital Discharges)	Gender/ Admin. data	TKR	receipt of procedure	In both 1990 and 2000, women had higher rates of TKR. Rates of TKR per 100,000 in 1990 were 30 for women compared to 23 in men, and in 2000 were 46 in women compared to 35 in men.
Olson; 2005[58]	1993-2001	Cross-sectional; Pop-based; N/A	Many; NR	Regional	W, B, H/ Admin. data	TKR	receipt of procedure	Connecticut hospital data (1996-1998) found that age adjusted rates per 100K discharges for TKR was highest for black women (115.8, 95% CI 103.9-127.7) and lowest for black men (44, 34.9-68.9) and Hispanic men (16.9, 10.1-23.8) and women (47.5, 37.8-57.2). White women had rates of 84.9 (82.4-87.4) and men 66.5 (63.9 -68.9).
Skinner; 2003[47]	1998-2000	Cross-sectional; Pop-based; N/A	403251; 0	National, Medicare	W, B, H/ Admin. data	TKR	receipt of procedure	Rate of TKA was higher for W women (5.97 procedures per 1000) than for H women (5.37 per 1000) and B women (4.84 per 1000). Rate for W men (4.82 procedures per 1000) was higher than H men (3.46 per 1000) and more than double that for B men (1.84 per 1000). The rates were lower for B men in nearly every region of the country (P<0.05). [For H population and for B women, racial/ethnic disparities were due in part to geographic differences rather than to differences in the rates for racial and ethnic groups within geographic areas. Residential segregation and low income levels contributed to disparities.]

45

A Comparison of Joint Replacement Disparities in VA and Non-VA Settings: A Systematic Review

Author; Date	Data Dates*	Study Type; Sample Selection; Response Rate/ Follow Up	Total pop; VA pop*	Data Source	Gender, Race**/ How determined	Joint Discussed***	Outcomes	Results
Escalante; 2002[48]	95-96	Cross-sectional; Pop-based; N/A	19311; 0	Medicare in NM, IL, TX, AZ	W, B, H, A/ Two or more sources	THR	receipt of procedure	1% THR recipients and 3.3% controls were H ($P < .001$). Odds of THR decreased as probability of H ethnicity increased (OR 1.00 non-H surnames to OR 0.36 H surnames (95% CI, 0.31, 0.43). Poverty did not modify the low odds of THR among H (OR, 0.25 Medicaid-eligible Hispanic persons; 95% CI, 0.19, 0.33; and OR, 0.30 Hispanic persons not Medicaid eligible; 95% CI, 0.24, 0.38).
Oishi; 1998[60]	85-89	Cross-sectional; NR; N/A	754; 0	Regional	W, A/ Medical record review	THR	receipt of procedure	THR for W was three to 25 times greater than that of Japanese, Chinese, Filipino, and Hawaiians. Risk of THR for W women was 4.4%, compared with 1.1% for Japanese women and 1.7% for Chinese women. For white men, the incidence rate is 3.6%, which is 4.5 to nine times greater than the rate for other ethnic groups. Some between region differences were noted (Hawaii versus San Francisco).
Giacomini; 1996[14]	1989-1990	Cross-sectional; Pop-based; N/A	6586; NR	OSHPD, regional	W, B, H, A/ NR	THR	receipt of procedure	Asians had higher odds of THR (OR 2.13 [95% CI 1.3-3.45]) than W. W had higher, but non-significant, odds of THR than H (OR 1.32 [.87-1.96]) and than B (OR 1.56 [.97-2.50]).
Katz; 1996[49]	85-90	Cross-sectional; Pop-based; N/A	414079; 0	Medicare, national	W, B/ Two or more sources	TKR	receipt of procedure	Odds of W receiving TKR were 1.5 times greater than for B. Adjusting for demographic factors, regional variation remained. TKR were over two and one-half times more likely for B women than for men (OR 1.66); the difference was only 24 percent for W women versus W men (OR = 1.24). Procedures were performed on W men much more often than on B, (OR 2.50). Difference between W and B women was much smaller (OR = 1.16).
Hoaglund; 1995[12]	84-88	Cross-sectional; Pop-based; N/A	1589; 0	San Francisco	W, B, H, A/ Medical record review	THR	receipt of procedure	The greatest annual rate of THR occurred in W women (97 per 100 000), followed by W men, B women, B men, H women, and H men. Smallest numbers were found in Asians, rate was 10% of W. Age standardized THR rates for primary coxarthrosis per 100 000 were greatest among W (43.0) and least among Asians (1.3 for Chinese). Mean age undergoing THR for primary coxarthrosis was 70 years for W and a decade younger in other groups.

Author; Date	Data Dates*	Study Type; Sample Selection; Response Rate/ Follow Up	Total pop; VA pop*	Data Source	Gender, Race**/ How determined	Joint Discussed***	Outcomes	Results
McBean; 1994[50]	86-92	Cross-sectional; Pop-based; N/A	a lot; 0	Medicare, national	W, B/ Admin. data	TKR, THR	receipt of procedure	TKR increased from 1986 and 1992, 98% among white beneficiaries and 121 percent among blacks. In 1992, the rate in blacks was 64% as great as for whites.
Wilson; 1994[11]	1980-1988	Cross-sectional; Pop-based; N/A	over 3000; NR	NHANES, Medicare	W, B/ Admin. data	TKR	receipt of procedure; Rate of OA	B were less often treated with TKR than W (men: OR=3.16 [1.69-5.91]; women: OR=1.55 [1.00-2.41]) for age 65-69.
Escarce; 1993[8]	1986	Cross-sectional; Pop based; N/A	1204022; 0	Medicare, national	W, B/ Admin. data	TKR, THR	receipt of procedure	W are two-fold more likely to undergo THR (RR 2.36 [1.92, 2.89]) or TKR (RR 2.02 [1.63, 2.49]) than blacks.

47

A Comparison of Joint Replacement Disparities in VA and Non-VA Settings: A Systematic Review

Key Question 2/ Generation 2 Evidence Table

Author; Date	Data Dates*	Study Type; Sample Selection; Response Rate/ Follow Up	Total pop; VA pop*	Data Source	Gender/ Race**/ How determined	Joint Discussed***	Outcomes	Results
Direct Comparison of VA and Non-VA Studies								
Ang; 2009[30]	2003–2006	Cohort/ Case-control; Convenience; 91.4%	676; 388	Single VA	W, B/ Self-reported	TKR, THR	Appropriateness, benefits, barriers, OA severity, length of time to referral; outcome expectations of surgery, perceived risk	Clinical appropriateness (HR 1.95, [95% CI] 1.15–3.32; $P <0.01$) predicted referral to orthopedic surgery. Neither race (HR 1.30, 95% CI 0.94–2.05; $P=0.1$) nor health beliefs (HR 1.0, $P = 0.5$) were associated with referral status.
Ang; 2009[31]	2003–2006	Cross-sectional; Convenience; 684/748	685; 388	Single VA	W, B/ Self-reported	TKR, THR	Appropriateness for procedure	There were no significant racial group differences ($p = 0.3$) in the proportions of those deemed clinically appropriate for TJR. Controlling for confounders (BMI, SES, education, county vs VA), race was not a predictor of clinical appropriateness for TJR (odds ratio 1.2, 95% CI [0.8–1.8], P =0.3).
Ang; 2008[32]	2003–2006	Cross-sectional; Convenience	691; 390	Single VA	W, B/ Self-reported	TJR	Benefits, barriers, OA severity, arthritis health, belief scale	B perceived less benefit from TJR than W (58.1 vs 44.3%; P=0.0001; OR=-60 (.42–.86), P=.005; B more likely to perceive barriers 42.4 vs 30.8%; P=.002; OR=.60, [CI] .42- .86, P=.005); Race not predictive of perceived severity of OA OR=.97 (.62–1.53), P=.9
VA Studies								
Hausmann 2011[29]	2005–2008	Cohort/ Case-control; Unclear; Not Specified	409; 409	VA	W, B/Self-reported	TKR, THR	Patient-provider communication	Visits with B, compared with W, contained less discussion of biomedical topics (B=-9.14, 95% CI -16.73 - -1.54) and more rapport-building statements (B=7.84; 95% CI 1.85- 13.82. No racial differences in length of visit, overall amount of dialogue, patient activation/engagement statements, discussions of psychosocial issues, physician verbal dominance, displays of positive affect, or evidence of informed decision making.

48

Author; Date	Data Dates*	Study Type; Sample Selection; Response Rate/ Follow Up	Total pop; VA pop*	Data Source	Gender/ Race**/ How determined	Joint Discussed***	Outcomes	Results
Hausmann; 2010[26]	2005-2008	Cohort/ Case-control; Unclear; Not specified	457; 457	VA	W, B/ Self-reported	TKR, THR	recommendation for procedure; receipt of procedure	Lower odds of receiving a TJR recommendation for B than W of similar age and disease severity (OR 0.46, [95% CI 0.26–0.83]; P=0.01). Difference was not significant adjusting for patient preference for TJR (OR 0.69, [95% CI 0.36–1.31], P=0.25).TJR less likely for B than W of similar age and disease severity (OR 0.41 [95% CI 0.16–1.0], P=0.06); difference reduced adjusting for recommendation for procedure at the index visit (OR 0.57 [95% CI 0.21–1.54], P=0.27).
Jones; 2008[33]	999	Cross-sectional; Convenience; N/A	939; 939	VA	W, B/ Self-reported	TKR, THR	prayer for pain, coping strategies, self efficacy	B more likely to perceive prayer helpful (OR 3.38, 95% CI [2.35 to 4.86]) and use prayer (OR 2.28, 95% [1.66 to 3.13]) to treat osteoarthritis pain as compared to W. B more likely to use coping and praying (β=0.74, 95% CI [0.50 to 0.99]).
Groeneveld; 2008[34]	2004-2006	Cross-sectional; Convenience; N/A	909; 909	VA	W, B/ Self-reported	TKR, THR	outcome expectations of surgery	B knee OA patients have lower expectation score (scale 0-76) than W even with adjustment for disease severity, SES, social support, literacy and trust (difference -3.8 points [95% CI 1.2, 6.3], and 4.2 points (95% CI 0.4, 8.0) among hip patients.
Weng; 2007[44]	999	Experimental; Convenience; Not specified	64; 64	VA	W, B/ Self-reported	TKR	outcome expectations of surgery, willingness to consider surgery, knowledge of surgery, alternative treatment	B had lower (but not significant) expectations for TKR than W for pain (WOMAC score 41 versus 34; P=0.18) and physical function (WOMAC score 38 versus 30; P = 0.13). B were less likely to have heard of TKR (49% versus 72%; P=0.02) and less likely to know someone who had TKR (34% versus 53%; P=0.05) than W.
Ibrahim; 2005[28]	1996-2000	Cohort/ Case-control; Pop-based; N/A	18811; 18811	NSQIP, VA	W, B, H/ Admin. data	TKR, THR	complications	Rates of non-infection and infection-related complications after TKA were higher among B compared with W (RR 1.50, [95% CI 1.08–2.10] and RR 1.42, [95% CI 1.06–1.90]). H had a higher risk of infection-related complications (RR 1.64, 95% CI 1.08–2.49) relative to W. Race/ethnicity was not associated with the risk of non-infection-related or infection-related complications for THR. 30-day mortality was 0.6% following TKA and 0.7% following THR, with no race/ ethnicity differences

A Comparison of Joint Replacement Disparities in VA and Non-VA Settings: A Systematic Review

Author; Date	Data Dates*	Study Type; Sample Selection; Response Rate/ Follow Up	Total pop; VA pop*	Data Source	Gender/ Race**/ How determined	Joint Discussed***	Outcomes	Results
Lopez; 2005[36]	1997-2000	Cross-sectional; Convenience; 728/770	596; 596	VA	W, B/ Self-reported	TKR, THR	participant/ provider relationship, perception access to care, receipt of referral	B were less likely than W to report difficulty getting medical care (OR 0.54 [0.34-0.88]). B were less likely than W to perceive the patient-physician relationship as excellent (24.7% vs. 36.3%, P<0.01) and less likely to have confidence in their primary physician (75.7% vs. 82.6%, P=0.04). Difficulty accessing care outside VA was not different between groups (52.4% vs. 52.2%, P=0.95).
Ang; 2003[37]	999	Cross-sectional; Convenience; 38 lost to follow up	558; 558	VA	W, B/ Self-reported	TKR, THR	perception of symptoms	B and W were not different in mean scores for WOMAC pain and WOMAC function when stratified by joint space narrowing, osteophyte and Kellgren Lawrence grades. After controlling for important covariates, ethnicity was not a significant predictor of WOMAC pain and function.
Ibrahim; 2003[38]	999	Cross-sectional; Convenience; Not specified	300; 300	VA	W, B/ Self-reported	TKR, THR	Perception of pain	B and W patients describe the quality of their chronic knee and hip pain differently. Chronic pain quality descriptions correlate with western Ontario and McMaster Universities Arthritis Index Scores but not radiologic stage of disease. {factor analyses}
Ibrahim; 2002[39]	1997-2000	Cross-sectional; Convenience; 738/776	596; 596	VA	W, B/ Self-reported	TKR, THR	willingness to consider surgery, outcome expecta-tions of surgery, familiarity with surgery	B were less likely than W to be willing to consider surgery for severe arthritis (OR 0.53, [95% CI 0.30-0.96]. After adjustment for outcome expectations, the difference between races in willingness to consider was not significant (OR 0.86, [95% CI 0.45-1.63]).
Ang; 2002[40]	97-00	Cross-sectional; Convenience; 95%	596; 596	VA	W, B/ Self-reported	TKR, THR	Role of prayer in the management of arthritis, willingness to consider surgery	B less willing than W to consider surgery for severe hip or knee arthritis pain (OR .059, [95% CI 0.34-0.99]). B more likely than W to perceive prayer as helpful in managing their arthritis (OR 2.1; [95% CI, 1.19, 3.72]).
Ibrahim; 2002[41]	97-00	Cross-sectional; Convenience; 738/776	596; 596	VA	W, B/ Self-reported	TKR, THR	QOL	For patients with chronic joint disease, B less likely than W to rate quality of life as excellent or very good. Difference persisted after adjusting for demographic, clinical, and psychosocial covariates, and severity of osteoarthritis (B=-0.121, P=.004).

Author; Date	Data Dates*	Study Type; Sample Selection; Response Rate/ Follow Up	Total pop; VA pop*	Data Source	Gender/ Race**/ How determined	Joint Discussed***	Outcomes	Results
Ibrahim; 2002[42]	97–00	Cross-sectional; Convenience; 738/776	596; 596	VA	W, B/ Self-reported	TKR, THR	outcome expectations of surgery, knowledge of joint replacement	B were less likely than W to have family/friends that had TJR (OR 0.39 [.26-.61]) or a good understanding of TRJ (OR 0.62 [.42-.92]). B more likely to expect longer hospital course (OR 4.09 [2.57-6.54]), moderate to extreme pain (OR 2.61 [1.74-3.89]), moderate to extreme difficulty walking after joint replacement (OR 2.76 [1.83-4.16]).
Ibrahim; 2001[43]	97–00	Cross-sectional; Convenience; 738/776	593; 593	VA	W, B/ Self-reported	joint replacement	efficacy arthritis treatment	B were more likely than W to perceive TJR as efficacious (OR .52 [.28-.98]) and more likely to rely on self-care measures for their arthritis (OTC meds: OR 1.76 [1.14-2.72]); friend/family advice: OR 2.11 [1.44-3.07]); decrease activities: OR 2.22 [1.28-3.85]); apply med cream: OR 2.27 (1.38-3.73]). Use of prayer more likely to be perceived as efficacious in B (OR 1.93 [1.19-3.14]).
Non-VA Studies								
Kamath; 2010[77]	2004	Cohort/ Case-control; Consecutive patients; Not specified	185; N/A	Single institution	B, Non-B/ Medical Record Review	TKR	outcome of procedure, outcome expectations of surgery	B men had longer delays to presentation than non B men (29.9 months [CI 17.2, 42.6] vs 20.0 months [CI 4.4, 35.6]) and worse 2-year KSS (89.6 months [CI 85.0, 94.2] vs 94.1 months [CI 91.2, 97.0]). B women had worse final ROM and similar final gains in ROM (postoperative minus preoperative) controlling for confounders.
Slover; 2010[78]	1997-2006	Cross-sectional; Consecutive patients; Not specified	3542; 0	Single institution	W, B, H/ Self-reported	TKR, THR	preop jt function	Lower function with Harris Hip Scores 4.9 (P< .0001) and 8.77 (P<.001) and Knee Society Scores that were 6.03 (P<.06) and 12.8 (P<.001) points lower in B and H patients than W.
Suarez-Almazor; 2010[73]	999	Qualitative; Unclear; Not specified	37, 0	Single institution	W, B, H/ Self-reported	TKR	willingness to consider surgery, outcome expectations of surgery, TKR Knowledge, Current prob knee OA	Attitudes and beliefs of surgical decision-making were primarily based on personal experiences. Personal experiences had both positive or negative impacts and included concerns about outcomes following surgery and possible complications. B did not have more concerns or fewer expectations.

A Comparison of Joint Replacement Disparities in VA and Non-VA Settings: A Systematic Review

Author; Date	Data Dates*	Study Type; Sample Selection; Response Rate/ Follow Up	Total pop; VA pop*	Data Source	Gender/ Race**/ How determined	Joint Discussed***	Outcomes	Results
Epstein; 2010[81]	2001-2004	Cross-sectional; Pop-based; Not specified	25598, 0	NYC discharge data	W, B, H, A/ Admin. data	THR	use HVH (hospital), use HVH (surgeon) receipt of procedure	B, Asians, H were more likely to be operated for TJR in low volume hospitals by low volume surgeons than whites (25.3%, 35.0%, 23.0% and 15.6%; P<.001)
Lavernia; 2010[74]	2000-2002	Cohort/ Case-control; Convenience; Not specified	331; 0	Single institution	W, B/ Self-reported	TKR, THR	outcome of procedure, fear of surgery, physical function	B patients had greater fear before joint arthroplasty compared with W. After surgery, B had higher fear subscale, cognitive subscale, and total PASS score (WOMAC physical function, pain, and total scores.
Berges; 2008[80]	2002-2003	Cohort/ Case-control; Pop-based; N/A	69793; NR	National	W, B, H, A/ Admin. data	THR	outcome of procedure	B and H had higher odds of discharge to home following hip replacement (B: OR 1.23 [1.107-1.41] and H: OR 1.5 [1.15-1.99]). B not significant. Men had higher odds of discharge to home (OR 1.18 [1.01-1.17]). Mean functional status change not predictive of discharge disposition (OR 1.10 [1.10-1.11])
Steel; 2008[62]	1998, 2000, 2002	Cohort/ Case-control; Pop-based; Not specified	14807; NR	National	W, B/ Self-reported	TKR, THR	need for surgery, receipt of procedure	Lower receipt of TJR in B (vs W: OR 0.47; CI 0.26-0.83) or less educated (0.65; 0.44-0.96). Differences not explained by employment, access, family responsibilities, disability, living alone, comorbidity, or excluding younger than Medicare.
Hanchate; 2008[57]	1994-2004	Cohort/ Case-control; Pop-based; Not specified	18439; NR	National	W, B, H/ Self-reported	TKR	receipt of procedure	B men (relative to W women) were less likely (OR 0.46 (0.28-0.78), [P < 0.05]) to receive TKA. Adjusting for economic factors, racial/ethnicity, TKA rates differences for women disappeared, while remaining large for B men (OR 0.56 [0.33-0.95]).
Kroll; 2007[76]	999	Qualitative; Convenience; Not specified	37; NR	Single institution	W, B, H/ Self-reported	TKR	attitudes and beliefs about TKR	Knee OA is experienced differently by ethnicity and groups, and perceptions of the cause of knee OA vary. Trust is important for H considering TKA. Economic factors do not constrain the decision to have surgery.

Author; Date	Data Dates*	Study Type; Sample Selection; Response Rate/ Follow Up	Total pop; VA pop*	Data Source	Gender/ Race**/ How determined	Joint Discussed***	Outcomes	Results
SooHoo; 2011[83]	1995-2005	Cross-sectional; Pop-based; N/A	138399; NR	OSHDD (California input database)	W, B, H, A/ Admin. data	THR	receipt by hospital volume	H had higher RRR [3.52 (95% [CI], 2.61-4.74; p < .001)] for the use of a low-volume hospital when compared to W. B (RRR, 1.78; p = .023) and Asian patients (RRR, 1.77; p = .048) also had a higher RRR compared to W for the use of low-volume hospitals
Liu; 2006[82]	2000-2004	Cross-sectional; Pop-based; N/A	1E+05; NR	OSHDD (California input database)	W, B, H, A/ Admin. data	TKR	receipt by hospital volume	B, Asians, and H were more likely to have TKR at low volume hospital than W (RR=1.32 [95% CI 1.25-1.39], RR=1.72 [95% CI 1.60-1.81], RR=1.64 [95% CI 1.58-1.69])
Byrne; 2006[84]	999	Cross-sectional; Random digit dialing; Not specified	391; NR	Single institution	W, B, H/ Self-reported	TKR	willingness to consider surgery	B less likely to chose surgery than W (OR 0.63 [CI 0.42, 0.93]). Women and older patients were also less likely to choose surgery (OR 0.69 [0.51, 0.94], OR 0.98 [0.97, 0.99]). Larger reductions in negative symptoms with surgery increased the likelihood of choosing surgery. No difference between the public and patients, and no effect of income level was noted.
Suarez-Almazor; 2005[69]	2001-2002	Cross-sectional; Pop-based; N/A	198; 0	Single institution	W, B, H/ Self-reported	TKR	recommendation for procedure, willingness to consider surgery, outcome expectations of surgery, preferences for surgery, familiarity of surgery	Physician more likely to discuss TKR with B (27%), 15% W, 11% H (P=.04). More W than minorities (B and H combined) considered TKR (42% vs 28%; P=.04). No differences between B, H, W being familiar with TKR.
Figaro; 2005[70]	999	Cross-sectional; Convenience; 104/114	94; 0	Harlem	B/ Self-reported	TKR	outcome expectations of surgery	In B with high rate of severe OA (mean QoL 7.6 ±1.7), few (36%) believed TKR would improve knee pain; and 45% felt surgery would not improve their health.
Byrne; 2004[85]	2001	Cross-sectional; Pop-based; 23%	193; 0	Harris County	W, B, H/ Self-reported	TKR	willingness to pay	Willingness to pay (WTP) as a percentage of income was lowest for B (16.7% for mild OA) as compared to 32.9% W, 26.4% H. Controlling for income, differences in WTP between B and W were significant in multivariate regression analyses, whereas values for H and W were not.

Author; Date	Data Dates*	Study Type; Sample Selection; Response Rate/ Follow Up	Total pop; VA pop*	Data Source	Gender/ Race**/ How determined	Joint Discussed***	Outcomes	Results
Figaro; 2004[71]	999	Qualitative; Convenience; Not specified	94; 0	Harlem	B/ Self-reported	TKR	outcome expectations of surgery, briefs and goals surgery, pref stay in current state, relationship w specialist	Content analyses identified 6 themes: preference for natural remedies, negative expectations of surgery, beliefs about God's control, preference for continuing in their current state, relationships with specialists, and fear of surgery or death.
Chang; 2004[72]	1998-1999	Qualitative; Consecutive; N/A	37; 0	Single institution	W, B/ Self-reported	TKR	concern about surgery	B women asked the most questions about criteria for TKR; W women asked about drawbacks from surgery; W men asked about devices; B men asked about financial issues and insurance coverage. Only W asked about intraoperative issues. W women asked about recuperation, functional recovery and pain, B women asked about long-term outcomes and support after surgery. W men asked about QOL and B men asked no questions. W men had greatest factual knowledge about surgery.
Ottenbacher; 2003[79]	1994-1998	Cross-sectional; Pop-based; N/A	12328; NR	4DSMR, national	W, B, H, A/ Two or more sources	TKR, THR	outcome of procedure	W and B were (P <0.05) more likely to be discharged home alone and responsible for their own care than Asian or H. 36% H after THA or TKA received inpatient medical rehabilitation 58% W, 67% B, and 56% Asians.
Blake; 2002[75]	999	Cross-sectional; Pop-based; 44%	970; 0	Medicare Manhattan	W, B/ Two or more sources	hip/knee surgery	Social network, Perception of benefit of arthritis treatment	42% B compared 65% W reported knowing someone who had surgery for hip or knee pain (P<.0001). B less likely that W to report that surgery had helped someone they knew with hip or knee pain (but not significant). B more likely to have sought care in ER/clinic 22% vs 9%, P<.005) and less likely to have seen an orthopedic surgeon 3% vs 15%, P<.0001). No racial differences in use of self-treatments (OTC, herbs PT, health/cold)

54

Author; Date	Data Dates*	Study Type; Sample Selection; Response Rate/ Follow Up	Total pop; VA pop*	Data Source	Gender/ Race**/ How determined	Joint Discussed***	Outcomes	Results
Wilson; 1994[11]	1980-1988	Cross-sectional; Pop-based; N/A	over 3000; NR	NHANES, Medicare	W, B/ Admin. data	TKR	receipt of procedure, Rate of OA	Prevalence of symptomatic OA knee was lower (but not significant) in W compared to B (men OR .39 [.13-1.14] and women OR .78 [.34-1.80]). Racial differences in TKR were consistent across income levels and were unexplained by B having operations at an earlier age or using competing procedures.

Key Question 3/ Generation 3 Evidence Table

Author; Date	Data Dates*	Study Type	Total pop; VA pop*	Data Source	Race**/ How determined	Joint Discussed***	Outcomes	Results
Weng; 2007[44]	999	Experimental; Convenience; Not specified	64; 64	VA	W,B/ Self-reported	TKR	Willingness to consider surgery, outcome expectations of surgery willingness to consider surgery, knowledge of surgery, alternative treatment	At baseline, 13% W and 29% B were willing to consider surgery (P<0.12); after intervention, 13% W and 33% B were willing to consider surgery (P<0.06).

*No data denoted as NR or 999

** W= White; B= Black; H= Hispanic; A=Asian

*** TKR=Total Knee Replacement; THR=Total Hip Replacement

www.ingramcontent.com/pod-product-compliance
Lightning Source LLC
Chambersburg PA
CBHW081615170526
45166CB00009B/2976